Current Issues in Healthcare

Health Improvement Programmes

Edited by

Salman Rawaf and Peter Orton

1 Wimpole Street, London W1M 8AE, UK
207 E Westminster Road, Lake Forest, IL 60045, USA
http://www.roysocmed.ac.uk

This book is published by the Royal Society of Medicine Services Ltd with financial support from the sponsor. The contributors are responsible for the scientific content and for the views expressed, which are not necessarily those of the sponsor, of the editors of the series or of the volume, of the Royal Society of Medicine or of the Royal Society of Medicine Press Ltd. Distribution has been in accordance with the wishes of the sponsor but a copy is available to any fellow of the Society at a privileged price.

British Library Cataloguing in Publication Data
A catalogue for this book is available from the British Library

ISBN 1-85315-388-5

Phototypeset by Techset Composition Limited, Salisbury, Wiltshire
Printed in Great Britain by Ebenezer Baylis, The Trinity Press, Worcester

List of Contributors

Dr Stuart Atkinson Principal Medical Advisor, PFIZER Ltd, London, UK

Ms Veena Bahl Department of Health Advisor on Minority Ethnic Health, UK

Dr Graham Bickler Director of Public Health, East Sussex, Brighton and Hove Health Authority, UK

Mr Andrew Boatswain Director of Solace Enterprises Ltd, Former Chief Executive, Swansea City Council, UK

Professor Robert Boyd Principal, St George's Hospital Medical School, London, UK

Ms Sarah Carr Research and Information Officer, The Implements Network, London, UK

Dr Vivien Chen Associate Director of Quality Assurance, Department of Health and Human Resources, Washington, USA

Dr Rachel Crowther Specialist Registrar in Public Health Medicine, Oxfordshire Health Athority, UK

Dr Anna Donald Clinical Lecturer, School of Public Policy, University College London and Royal Free Medical Schools, London, UK

Mr Norman Evans Pharmaceutical Advisor, Merton, Sutton and Wandsworth Health Authority, London, UK

Mr Gary Fereday Association of Community Health Councils for England and Wales, London, UK

Mrs Sue Gallagher Chief Executive, Merton, Sutton and Wandsworth Health Authority, London, UK

Professor Hamid Ghodse Professor of Addictive Behaviour, St George's Hospital Medical School, London, UK

Mr Philip Grant Head of Healthcare Commissioning Development, NHS Executive, Department of Health, Leeds, UK

Professor Andrew Haines Department of Health and Epidemiology, University College London and Royal Free Medical Schools, London, UK

Dr Nicholas R Hicks Consultant in Public Health Medicine, Oxfordshire Health Authority, UK

Professor Rachel Jenkins Professor of Psychiatry, WHO Collaborating Centre, Institute of Psychiatry, London, UK

Mr Gerald Jones Chief Executive, Wandsworth Borough Council, London, UK

Dr Owen Keyes-Evans Senior Registrar in Public Health Medicine, Merton, Sutton and Wandsworth Health Authority, London, UK

Dr Azim Lakhani Director, National Centre for Health Outcomes Development, London School of Hygiene and Tropical Medicine, London, and Institute of Health Sciences, Oxford, UK

Mrs Fiona Marshall Specialist Nurse and Business Manager, Department of Addictive Behaviour and Psychological Medicine, St George's Hospital Medical School, London, UK

Dr Peter Orton Senior Lecturer, Institute of General Practice, University of Exeter, Exeter, and General Practitioner, Hatfield Heath, UK

Professor Leon Polnay Professor of Community Paediatrics, University of Nottingham, Nottingham, UK

Dr Kelly Powell Specialist Registrar in Public Health Medicine, Merton, Sutton and Wandsworth Health Authority, London, UK

Dr Salman Rawaf Director of Clinical Standards/Senior Lecturer, Merton Sutton and Wandsworth Health Authority, London, UK

Dr Timothy Riley Head of Clinical Outcomes and Effectiveness, Public Health Development Unit, NHS, Leeds, UK

Dr Geoff Roberts Chairman, Surrey Heath Primary Care Group and General Practitioner, Camberley, Surrey, UK

Professor Andrew Stevens Professor of Public Health and Head of Department, The University of Birmingham, Birmingham, UK

Dr Geraldine Strathdee Consultant Psychiatrist, Institute of Psychiatry, London, UK

Professor Anthea Tinker Professor of Social Gerontology, King's College London and President Section of Geriatrics and Gerontology, Royal Society of Medicine, London, UK

▶The Editors

Salman Rawaf is a Director of Clinical Standards and Consultant Public Health Physician for Merton, Sutton and Wandsworth Health Authority and Senior Lecturer in Public Health Medicine at St George's Hospital Medical School, London. He has been a District Medical Officer and Director of Public Health in Merton and Sutton since 1988, with wide experience in health policy, disease management and clinical standards. He is both consultant and advisor for the World Health Organization and other bodies and has served on many national and international committees. Recently, he has co-edited *Assessing Health Needs* published jointly by the Royal College of Physicians and the Department of Health. He is a member of the Board of the Faculty of Public Health Medicine and co-edits the continuing professional development journal *Public Health Medicine*.

Peter Orton is a general practitioner at Hatfield Heath in Essex. He works in a rural dispensing practice that participates in general practitioner training and national morbidity surveillance. His medical interests include medical education, stress in general practitioners, the use of management in practice, auditing performance and healthcare system comparisons. He is a Senior Lecturer in the Institute of General Practice at Exeter University and in the Department of Continuing Education at Bath University. He is Past President of the Section of General Practice at the Royal Society of Medicine. His numerous publications include *Primary care: Who leads?* Lancet annual review (1996) and *Stress in Family Physicians; Solutions and Strategies* Canadian Family Physician (1995). He has written or contributed to three books: *Reviving Primary Care: a US-UK comparison* (Radcliffe), *UK Health Care: the facts* (Kluwer) and *GP's Management Handbook* (Saunders).

Acknowledgements

The Editors are grateful to Pfizer Limited, The Department of Health and Merton Sutton and Wandsworth Health Authority for their contribution to the running costs of the December 1998 Royal Society of Medicine symposium on which this book is based, and to the production costs of the book. Special thanks go to Wendy Meynell of Merton Sutton and Wandsworth Health Authority for her administrative support and to the Royal Society of Medicine Press for agreeing to publish. Mostly, we would like to thank all our colleagues for their time, efforts and contributions and our families for their patience and tolerance.

Contents

Foreword

One of the leading roles of the Royal Society of Medicine is its academic programme, which is designed to explore the frontiers of developments in medical care. I was delighted to lead and participate in the academic and professional day of discussion on which this book is based. The expert groups involved focused on the health improvement programme (HImP)—the cornerstone of the white paper *The New NHS: Modern and Dependable* on the proposed changes in the NHS.

I first understood the practical difficulties of introducing health improvement policies when I was District General Manager of Oxfordshire Health Authority in the early 1980s. Here, at the joint consultative committee between the county council, voluntary agencies and the health authority, there was often a failure of common purpose and agreeing who would pay the revenue consequences of any proposed initiative often proved too great a hurdle. In spite of this, some good things were done.

Then, we had the national initiative of the *Health of the Nation*. An enormous amount of evidence-gathering and structure for implementation and monitoring went into this and some really important lessons were learned. Although accusations were made that such a scheme smacked too much of the 'nanny sate', I believe it did add impetus to the way we influence our lifestyle (eg the drive to reduce cigarette smoking) and focused public attention quite effectively on the five target areas. As a side-benefit, but under its general umbrella, it demonstrated exciting and very important health variations, although the rigid structure of the *Health of the Nation* could not tackle these. We shall have to see whether or not its successor, *Our Healthier Nation*, will achieve more: it is, of course, much too soon to tell.

HImPs are our endeavour to bring about health gain by tackling the well-known causes of ill health. They are to be locally established by co-ordination of the relevant agencies and the public's aspiration. They are three-year programmes and will be subjected to evaluation, particularly of their impact on the local population's health. I believe the idea is a good one, but if it is to deliver, it will need to be set going and monitored with extreme care. Otherwise, much money could be spent and people's time taken up and expectations raised without a useful outcome.

The Royal Society of Medicine's endeavour and this book on the millennium approach to health and healthcare is most welcome. Experts in the field have identified the best approaches to HImP implementation, monitoring and evaluation based on scientific evidence and experience, with specific disease and care group examples. This book will be a great asset to health authorities and primary care groups as commissioners of health, to primary care teams, hospitals, community service managers and practitioners as providers of healthcare and to all those interested in the ways and means of improving the health of their nation and communities.

Sir Christopher Paine
Immediate Past President, Royal Society of Medicine, London

Foreword

▶ Introduction

Improving health is the ultimate goal of any health service, irrespective of the source of funding. But individuals' and population health are usually determined by many factors, most of which are outside the control of the health services. Some are also beyond the control of the individual and require action from government and society: air pollution, poverty, low income, unemployment, and poor housing, for example, are at least as important as individual lifestyle factors[(1)].

Nearly all sections of society in the Western world have benefited from a steady decrease in mortality rates from most diseases and a significant increase in life expectancy during the course of this century. However, systematic variations in mortality rates between different groups and geographical areas have been observed in the UK and other Western countries consistently. Indeed, there are marked differences according to occupational class, sex, region and ethnicity, in life expectancy, healthy life status and incidence and survival from a range of diseases[(2–4)]. In developing countries, the picture is much worst and, in many places, people are struggling for survival.

Many governments across the world are concerned about such variations in health and are trying to invent and adopt the best possible means of addressing them. The UK Government, for example, as part of its modernization programmes in all aspects of public life and services, has adopted the concept of *Health Improvement Programmes* (*HimPs*) for the *New NHS*[(5)]. HimPs are to be the means by which the health services, local governments and all partners in health are to plan and act in an integrated and comprehensive way to improve the health of the population overall and provide the highest standards of healthcare for those who need it. These parties will be held accountable for such measurable improvement.

Developing, implementing and monitoring health improvement programmes is a task requiring not just expertise and specific skills, but also the ability to cut across organizational boundaries, to look at things differently, to be flexible, to tackle difficult issues rather than avoiding them and, above all, to pool all available resources (human and financial). The authors of the 20 chapters and two appendices that follow decant the theories and practical experiences involved in developing, implementing and monitoring HImPs.

Chapter 1 sets the national perspective, Chapters 2 and 3, while reflecting on the last 50 years of the National Health Service, propose various possible approaches to improving health through learning from past experience and re-evaluating the current practical approaches to healthcare needs assessment. HImP implementation will challenge all partners and Chapters 4–7 highlight this through the experiences of a health authority chief executive, a general practitioner, a consultant and a local authority chief executive. Chapter 6, in particular, focuses on the difficult issue of influencing change in clinical behaviour and suggests 10 practical steps towards implementing such change.

One of the key elements for the success of the development and implementation of an effective HImP is to involve the local population (not just the users) and to take account of their perspectives. Chapter 8 gives an account of the role of the Community Health Councils and proposes a range of public involvement and consultation methods. Ensuring that quality is at the heart of health service planning and delivery is not a simple task and we have devoted three chapters (9–11) to addressing clinical standards, clinical quality and outcomes, simultaneously building on experiences from both sides of the Atlantic. Increasing the ability, professional skills and skill-mix of health professionals so that they may work better in partnership with the public is paramount and Chapter 12 outlines the quadruple roles of higher medical and health professionals' education and how to achieve a balance between research and education on one hand and service innovation and provision for the local wider community on the other.

The last quarter of this century has seen the greatest technical advances in human history and more is to come as we enter the millennium. While technology has impacted heavily on individuals and society in general, it has probably had its biggest impact on the ways in which we maintain health, deliver healthcare and intervene with the ill health of the human body. The benefits may be obvious, but the costs and risks are not yet fully assessed; however, such technologies still enter the NHS at a speed many health planners and policy makers find difficult to cope with. Chapter 13 identifies the challenging methods for evaluating and managing the entry of new therapies and technologies into the health service—a process which is likely to have significant financial and clinical impact.

While a local HImP should be able to address any significant health and healthcare issues in which improvement is possible, we have limited ourselves to three major disease areas and three care groups (Chapters 14–19). The chapter on coronary heart disease describes a tool for the development and implementation of a HImp, based on the collective experience of nine district health authorities. The chapter on mental illness demonstrates practical steps towards addressing the substantial inequality in its distribution, related services and their outcomes. The chapter on substance use and misuse suggests practical steps towards developing a HImP to tackle drug misuse—a problem that is not only widespread but the number one public health problem in many western countries.

Some people from minority ethnic groups have specific health and social needs and HImPs provide an opportunity to address these as part of the mainstream agenda, as chapter 17 describes. The key to successful population health in the future is through young people laying good foundations for health early in life today. Chapter 18 identifies the main areas in which child health could be improved and how to address the positive and negative influences on children's health in the locality. Chapter 19 addresses the health of the expanding population of older people. Promoting and maintaining good health in, as well as tackling the multiple pathology that characterizes, older people is one of the HImPs more important roles. Finally, chapter 20 gives an overview of the HImP approach, looking at its strengths and weaknesses and the way forward for such a long-term commitment to health improvement.

Partnership is an essential ingredient for any successful HImP; that is, in ensuring that HImPs are *specific*, *measurable*, *achievable*, *resourced and time-bound* (*SMART*). The main challenge that HImPs currently set is to move from the current *fragmented approaches* to health improvement to an *integrated approach*. Central to their success, therefore, is long-term commitment, continued investment, the achievement of a careful balance between prevention and treatment, and perseverance. In particular, the long-term commitment is a challenge, particularly in those countries in which demand fa· exceeds supply, in which political priorities are usually short-term, and whose individual citizens are less willing to take responsibility for their own health improvement.

We hope that this book with its theoretical frameworks and practical experiences will help politicians, policy makers, planners, health professionals and social workers, among others, to work in a collaborative and integrated way towards the development, implementation and measurement of their local HImPs.

References

1 Secretary of State for Health. *Saving lives: Our Healthier Nation.* London: The Stationery Office, 1999.

2 Department of Health. *Variations in health: what can the Department of Health and the NHS do?* London: DoH, 1995.

3 Rawaf S, Bahl V. *Assessing health needs of people from minority ethnic groups.* London: Royal College of Physicians, 1998.

4 Acheson D (Chairman). *Independent inquiry into inequalities in health.* London: The Stationery Office, 1998.

5 Secretary of State for Health. *The New NHS: Modern, Dependable.* London: The Stationery Office, 1997.

Drs Salman Rawaf and Peter Orton
Director of Clinical Standards/Senior Lecturer, Merton, Sutton and Wandsworth Health Authority, London, and Senior Lecturer, Institute of General Practice, University of Exeter, Exeter and General Practitioner, Hatfield Heath, UK

▶1

National perspective

Mr Philip Grant
Head of Healthcare Commissioning Development, NHS Executive,
Department of Health, Leeds, UK

Nearly all sections of society in the Western world have benefited from a steady decrease in mortality rates from most diseases and significant increase in life expectancy during this century[1]. However, systematic variations in mortality rates between different groups and geographical areas have consistently been observed in the UK and elsewhere[1]. Indeed, over the years the Chief Medical Officers' annual reports of the state of public health have shown that in the UK there are marked differences by occupational class, sex, region and ethnicity in life expectancy, healthy life status and incidence of and survival from a range of diseases[1,2].

The consultative document *Our Healthier Nation*[3] published two months after the white paper *The New NHS: Modern and Dependable*[4] had two specific aims.

- To improve the health of the population as a whole by increasing the length of people's lives and the number of years people spend free of illness
- To improve the health of the worst off in society and to narrow the health gap.

These could be achieved through partnership between government, local communities and individuals to improve everybody's health through specific health improvement programmes (HImPs)[3].

HImPs, according to the white paper, will be an effective vehicle for making a major and sustained impact on health problems of every locality in the country'. All these programmes 'taken together will form a concentrated national programme to improve health and tackle inequalities'[4].

National priorities

The Government's and its Department of Health's key main aim is 'to reduce the incidence of avoidable illness, disease and injury in the population'. This will be achieved through the following key objectives:

- to treat people will illness, disease or injury quickly and effectively on the basis of need alone
- to enable people who are unable to perform essential activities of daily living, including those with chronic illness, disability or terminal illness, to live as full and normal lives as possible
- to maximize the social development of children in stable family settings.

The Government will modernize services to meet these objectives by:

- tackling the root causes of ill health
- breaking down the barriers between services

- ensuring uniformly high-quality standards and maximizing value for money
- making services faster and more convenient.

To achieve these aims and objectives the Government has proposed a local systematic approach to improve the health of the population—the HImP.

What is a HImP?

A HImP, therefore, will be the local strategy for improving *health* and *healthcare*. It will be the means to deliver national targets in each health authority area. The health authority will have lead responsibility for drawing up the HImP in consultation with NHS trusts, primary care groups, other primary care professionals such as dentists, opticians and pharmacists, the public and other partner organizations[(4)].

These HImPs, as well as looking at the overall health of the local population, will also focus action on people who are socially excluded and need the most support in getting back on their feet.

The local HImP will cover the:

- most important *health* needs of the local population and how these are to be met by the NHS and its partner organizations through broader action on public health
- main *healthcare requirements* of local people and how local services should be developed to meet them either directly by the NHS or where appropriate jointly with social services
- *range, location and investment required in local health services* to meet the needs of local people.

Duty of real partnership

Many factors influence an individual's and population's health. A good number of these are beyond the control of the individual and require action from government and society—air pollution, poverty, low income, unemployment, poor housing and crime and disorder are as, if not more, important as individual lifestyles[(3)].

Thus, in developing, implementing and measuring the impact of such local strategy for improving health, health authorities should work in partnership with a wide range of local interests, including local authorities, to tackle the social, economic and environmental roots of ill health. Such partnership will be under a new *statutory duty* placed on local NHS bodies to work together for the common good. This will extend to local authorities, strengthening the existing requirements under the 1997 NHS Act. Furthermore, the Government intends to place on local authorities a duty to promote the economic, social and environmental wellbeing of their areas[(4)].

The HImP process

The white paper and subsequent health circulars have made clear that the HImP process should:

- bring *together* the local NHS with local authorities and others, including the voluntary sector, to set the strategic framework for improving health, tackling inequalities and developing faster, more convenient services of a consistently high standard

- be *action focused*, setting out high-level objectives and a summary of the commitments of the local players to deliver these
- include *measurable targets* for improvement[5]
- show that the action proposed is *based on evidence* of what is known to work
- show what *measure of local progress* will be used
- indicate which organizations have been *involved in drawing up the plan*, what their *contribution* will be and how they will be held to *account* for delivering it
- ensure that the plan is *easy to understand* and *accessible to the public*
- be a vehicle for setting strategies for shaping local health services.

Systematic components

The HImP should be seen as a systematic process which includes the following:

- *Health and needs assessment:* brings the partners together to pool their knowledge of the health and needs of the community they jointly serve
- *Shared vision:* develops a shared statement of the local response to national priorities (eg Our Healthier Nation) and those set in response to local needs, including action to tackle inequalities
- *Set objectives:* sets clear, specific and measurable objectives for health and healthcare improvement and records the commitments of various local players
- *Identify resources:* identifies targets and milestones and sets the resource framework for the NHS and for health and social care
- *Measure outcomes:* in the light of the objectives, sets, assesses and measures the objectives achieved (effectiveness of the programme), highlights difficulties and obstacles and shares success and good practices.

Wider context of HImP

HImPs should be underpinned by:

- cross-referencing to relevant standards of local authority plans (eg housing, transport, etc)
- plans of other non-NHS partners
- detailed healthcare strategies
- long-term service arrangements
- infrastructure plans addressing workforce, capital and information needs across the whole health and social care system
- service and financial frameworks.

The first HImPs

Detailed guidance has been issued[5] and requires every health authority to lead the local development of HImPs by April 1999. Initial HImPs will cover a three-year rolling timeframe with part of the programme reviewed in depth each year. However, it has been recognized from the beginning that it will take time to develop fully HImPs that involve all local interests. A key priority for the first year must be to build and strengthen local partnership arrangements.

The first HImPs beginning in 1999/2000 are not expected to be comprehensive. They should aim to tackle a selected number of national and local issues while setting out the action planned to develop a full HImP for 2000/1 and a comprehensive HImP for 2002/3. Such a programme will need to cover the priorities set out in the National Priorities Guidance, the four *Saving Lives: Our Healthier Nation* priority areas[(6)] and action on local inequalities.

Each HImP will also incorporate joint investment plans (JIP) between health authorities and social services departments as detailed in *Better Services for Vulnerable People*[(7)]. For 1999/2000 JIPs will consider the needs of older people and one more locally agreed vulnerable group.

Consultation and involvement

For any HImP to be successful from the stage of inception to full implementation, it should be developed in full consultation with and involvement of the community and its organized groups. It is therefore essential that the health authority should secure the widest possible active involvement of statutory and non-statutory organizations and the public at large. It is a requirement for the HImP to be published and to contain a statement on who has been involved in its preparation and how. Views should be sought regularly to inform the annual rolling programme and a separate consultation, as now, on proposals for significant service changes, closure or reconfigurations should be sought.

Conclusions

HImPs will be effective vehicles for achieving a sustained impact on the health problems of every locality in the country. As well as addressing the overall health needs and status of the local population, they will also focus action on people who are socially excluded and need the most support in getting back on their feet. For any HImP to succeed in achieving its objectives, a comprehensive and detailed health needs assessment, joint vision, real partnership, clear measurable objectives, plan for action and proper monitoring process are needed. The collective HImPs across the country should form a concentrated national programme to improve health and tackle health inequalities for a healthier nation.

Key messages

- The HImP is the local strategy to improve health and healthcare
- The health authority will have lead responsibility for the HImP (developing, implementing and monitoring)
- HImPs should be developed and implemented in real partnership (sharing vision, resources and expertise)
- HImPs will initially cover a three-year rolling programme
- Public, statutory and non-statutory organizations should be fully involved
- Primary care groups and teams will have a key role in the development and implementation of the action-focused, measurable, local HImP.

References

1 Department of Health. *Variations in health: what can the Department of Health and the NHS do?* A report of Sub-Group of the Chief Medical Officer's Health of the Nation Working Group. London: DoH, 1995.

2 Chief Medical Officers (England, Scotland, Wales, Northern Ireland). *On the state of public health.* London: The Stationery Office, 1990–1998.

3 Secretary of State for Health. *Our healthier nation: a contract for health.* London: The Stationery Office, 1998.

4 Secretary of State for Health. *The new NHS: modern and dependable.* London: The Stationery Office, 1997.

5 NHS Executive. *Health improvement programmes: planning for better health and better healthcare.* Health Service Circular 1998/167. Leeds: NHSE, 1998.

6 Secretary of State for Health. *Saving Lives: Our Healthier Nation.* London: The Stationery Office, 1999.

7 Department of Health. *Better services for vulnerable people.* London: The Stationery Office, 1998.

▶2

Approaches to health improvement programmes

Dr Salman Rawaf

Director of Clinical Standards/Senior Lecturer, Merton Sutton and Wandsworth Health Authority, London, UK

Dr Peter Orton

Senior Lecturer, Institute of General Practice, University of Exeter, Exeter, and General Practitioner, Hatfield Heath, UK

The National Health Service (NHS) was created in 1948 against a background of success in tackling some of the major diseases of the day (sexual diseases, acute illnesses) and technological advances. There were also marked improvements in many public health areas such as sanitation, water supply, housing, nutrition and control of many communicable diseases[(1,2)]. All of this generated high expectations among the British public for better health and healthcare and prolonged life. Weary of such expectations, the founders of the NHS hoped that reducing the ill health of the population as a whole would diminish the need for healthcare. While their optimistic dream was soon established as a mirage, the service continued to increase on the basis of rapid medical advances, which, in turn, continued to generate higher expectations and more demands[(3,4)]. These were compounded by the accompanying demographic changes—an increased population of older people and, inevitably, chronic diseases. The NHS drifted away from its main goal of improving the population's health, and into a 'sickness' service drawing wide criticism from all sides.

The first explicit attempt by the government to provide a strategic approach to improving the overall health of the population, *The Health of the Nation* (*HOTN*), was launched in 1992[(5)]. For nearly six years, this was the central plank of health policy in England. Accumulating huge management costs, however, it failed, over its short life-span, to realize its potential. HOTN was also handicapped from the outset by numerous flaws—both conceptual and procedural[(6)].

The new Labour administration that came to power in 1997 wasted no time, as part of their modernization programmes, in initiating one of the major reforms the NHS had seen since its inception[(7)]. *Our Healthier Nation: a contract for health*[(8)] included a new strategy for health: After a consultative period of 18 months, a follow-up government white paper *Saving Lives: Our Healthier Nation* was published and described by the Prime Minister as 'a significant step towards better health'[(9)].

The key questions with respect to the improvement of public health and healthcare provision are currently What do we mean by health? and What are the possible ways of improving the health of the population?

This chapter will address the concept of health, what we have learnt from the past 50 years about improving it, and, bearing these two in mind, the possible approaches to health improvement and what each means to the various stakeholders involved, each of whom perceives health and health issues differently.

The concept of health

Definitions of health have ranged from the simple absence of disease to the many comprehensive notions of wellbeing expressed by different communities and cultures[10]. Health can be described in medical terms (ie biological, the absence of a defined illness), or in social terms (ie functional, the departure from normal physiological function). The World Health Organization (WHO) defines health in a more holistic way, as 'a state of complete physical, mental, social and "spiritual" wellbeing'. This idealistic and holistic concept of health is far-removed from the experiences of most human beings. A person's lifestyle and health is, in fact, determined not only by personal factors such as genetics, race and culture, but also, and at least as importantly, by social, economic, environmental and political influences[10–12].

Thus, there is no uniformly accepted definition of health. Health and illness are not only highly subjective terms, but may carry different meanings in different cultures and social classes. Indeed, with new discoveries and advancement in medical knowledge, the concepts of health and illness are changing over time. We have seen, alongside the relatively recent information revolution, for example, raised patient expectations and the development of a conviction among many that nothing is beyond the reach of doctors and modern medicine. The assumption on the part of the patient that whatever problem they have can be translated into a diagnostic category and therefore dealt with by their doctor has further increased demands on an already stretched service.

Since 'health' is a highly subjective term influenced by some or all the factors mentioned above, measuring improvements in it can probably, therefore, only be achieved using high-level indicators such as morbidity and mortality data

Learning from experience

Lessons from fifty years' experience of the British NHS

The good: a success story

Despite major economic and social changes over the past five decades, the NHS is still operating under its founding principles. It is:

- free at the time of delivery
- comprehensive
- attempting equality in provision
- defining itself within acceptable standards.

It has not only contributed, beyond compare, to the improvement in the UK population's health, but has managed to sustain many organizational changes, including the introduction of the quasi-market in 1990. Despite frequent criticism of wastage and ineffective resource use, it has proved efficient in its operation. Indeed, the unit cost has decreased steadily since 1948[1]. Effectively encompassing most of the very many medical advances it has witnessed, its healthcare protocols have continuously changed and developed.

The bad: a national sickness service

Having dealt competently with most infectious diseases, most of the conditions the NHS currently handles are those relating to chronic illness and ageing, and that are the consequences of individuals' behaviours and lifestyles. With the fuelled expectations already discussed, the focus of the service has moved further and further towards treating illness rather than promoting health and preventing ill-health. Many now perceive the NHS to be an 'illness' service, paying less attention to real partnership with the many public and voluntary sector organisations interested in promoting the 'bigger health picture' and focusing on the more global determinants of health (eg housing, pollution, employment, wealth, politics).

The ugly: wide variations in health, healthcare and clinical standards

Despite a steady improvement in health in general, 'too many are still unnecessarily falling ill and dying sooner than they should'[(8)]. There are still wide variations in health, between individuals and groups of individuals. Mortality rates in different groups of the population have varied consistently, for example[(13)]. Not just life expectancy, but lifestyle and the incidence of and survival from a range of diseases differ markedly according to occupational class, gender, region and ethnicity, in most industrialised countries[(13)]. Indeed, 'the gap in health between those at the top and bottom of the social class scale has widened'[(14)].

Although the NHS provides excellent coverage in terms of prevention, primary care and secondary care (including specialist services), there are still wide variations in access to and the quality of these services. These variations in healthcare provision can be attributed to many factors, but the most important is the way in which services evolved historically. Very few services are based on need; instead, most are shaped through demand and professional leadership. Thus, the less demanding populations (those lower on the social scale, and ethnic groups, etc) have been marginalized. An 'inverse care law' still exists, for example in primary care provision, especially in the inner cities[(14,15)] and there is a 'lottery of treatment' for cancer patients and those requiring other highly specialist services[(16)]. Variations in the funding of some interventions (for example: in-vitro fertilization, dementia, substance misuse, care of older people, gender change) by health authorities have been widely reported.

In fact, one of the 'ugliest faces' of the NHS is the tolerance of the medical professions of such variations in clinical practice, standards and outcomes[(17)]. This issue has been highlighted by a number of well-publicised serious failures in clinical care and the Inquiries that followed—the Bristol paediatric cardiothoracic deaths, for example, and the problems experienced in the breast and cervical cancer screening programmes. Such variations are not just seen between regions, but between smaller localities within a region. Local data on variations in treatment are interesting but worrying.

Prevention of further cardiac events in post-myocardial infarction patients can be used to explore the variations issue further. Current knowledge shows that a combination of lipid-lowering agents, aspirin and changes in lifestyle can prevent further major cardiac events in this group of patients. Twenty-five patients need to be treated with aspirin for a year in order to prevent one myocardial infarction or death (the number needed to treat or NNT is therefore 25), and similar findings are reported in relation to lipid lowering agents (statins). Yet, as Figures 2.1 and 2.2 illustrate, there are very large variations in the prescription of these agents in general practice after discharge from hospital [unpublished data: Rawaf S, Evans N, Seyan R, Floyd K]. This is an example of where audit can be applied to quality of care using an evidence-based approach. Referrals to secondary care (diagnostic and/or interventional; for example, referral to endoscopy for dyspepsia patients) are quite variable—even within a small locality and to the same hospital—despite the publication of national and local guidelines.

Lessons from the 1990 reforms

Change is part and parcel of any modern organisation. While the NHS has been exposed to many changes since its inception in 1948, those instigated in 1990 have been the most dramatic[(18)]. Many factors have been identified as contributary causes for such reforms: efficiency drives, increased demands on services, and political dogma. The latter was very significant in the 1980s and culminated in the 1990 reforms, designed to bring a distinctive set of political ideas to the public sector services[(19)]. Thus, the 'quasi-market' was born, with all the problems associated with such an approach in the public sector. Following the reforms, the 1990–97 NHS was seen as:

- Provider-led: with the illusion of 'competition' providers moved away from the public health agenda ('a sickness service')
- Having fragmented services: health organizations within the NHS, once again in the spirit of competition, moved away from any meaningful partnerships to identify and

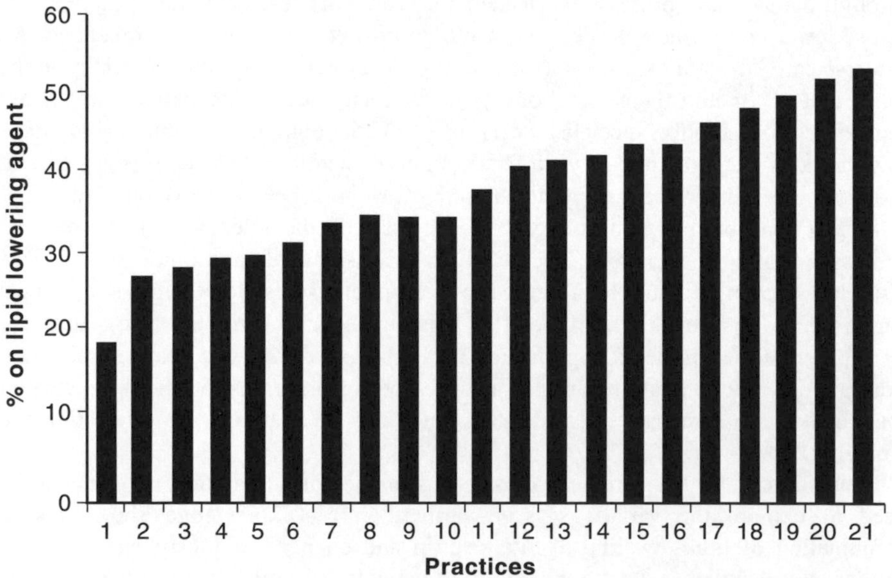

Fig. 2.1 Percentage of post-myocardial infarction patients prescribed a lipid-lowering agent (statin/fibrate) according to practice, South London, 1999.

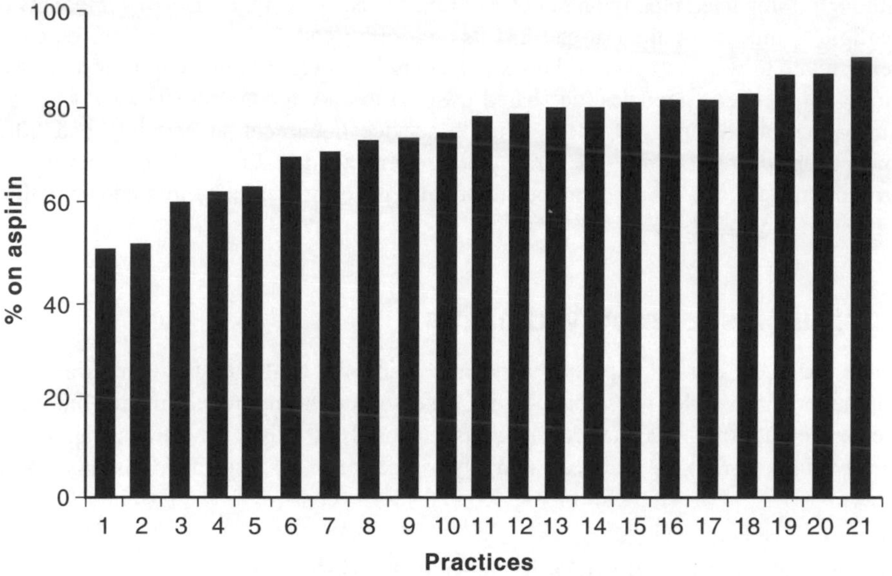

Fig. 2.2 Percentage of post-myocardial infarction patients on aspirin according to practice, South London, 1999.

meet the needs of the population ('chinese wall syndrome'). A craze for new logos characterized this period

- Having a two-tiered system: to help ensure that the reforms were successful, the demands of fundholding primary care practices were prioritized. Eager to attract funds, hospital and community trusts prioritized fundholding patients and also provided a range of previously untested methods of service delivery (eg outreach clinics). Many people were uncomfortable with this partisan approach to healthcare ('lottery of provision') in their national public health service
- Centralized: many felt that the reforms strengthened 'command and control' within the system, with more accountability to the centre of control ('feeding the beast'). Lack of democracy within the NHS meant that many priorities were set nationally, and in response to political agendas rather than local needs
- having lapsed clinical standards: in attempts to win the lion's share of the 'market', there was more focus on quantity than quality of service (eg in the Bristol case).

Lessons from the Health of the Nation

The *Health of the Nation* was published in 1992 as the first explicit strategy to improve the health of the population of England as a whole[5]. Based on the WHO's *Health for All*, similar strategies were published for other parts of the UK. The *Health of the Nation* focused on five major public health problems: coronary heart disease and stroke, cancer, mental health, accidents and sexual health. Its objectives were clear and it was welcomed, widely, both within and outside the NHS. However, *The Health of the Nation* failed, over its five-year life-span, to realize its full potential[6]. It was handicapped from the outset by numerous conceptual and procedural flaws and, although it impacted clearly on policies during the early years, by 1997 its impact was negligible. Indeed, by then, it had lost its credibility and priorities were, once again, being given to waiting lists and books balancing[(6)]. There was no central or local co-ordination between agencies, no shared ownership and, for many, *The Health of the Nation* became simply yet another health service document. It certainly had little impact on primary care: 'General practitioners tended to focus on the health promotion aspects of their contracts alone, and gave little priority to strategic action for health beyond this'[(6)].

Approaches to improved health

There are many possible approaches to improving the health of individuals and the population as a whole. These include the 'disease-burden' approach (medical model), the 'socio-environmental' approach (holistic model) and the 'educational' approach (behavioural model). In practice, we apply a mixture of all three and, possibly, some others.

The disease-burden approach (medical model)

This approach is based on the concept that individuals can define the burden that their illnesses place on them and, through preventive and early intervention(s), are able to reduce this burden on themselves and society. Within this model, the biological, physiological and social causes of the disease and its contributing risk factors are easier to define. Intervention(s) at primary and secondary prevention levels can be identified and categorized (Figure 2.3). The individuals take most of the responsibility for action to improve their health, but society helps and supports those who need it. The disease-burden approach fits well with current medical practices and education but, above all, it makes it easier to measure intervention outcome(s), many of which

Category of intervention	Examples
Prevention of risk factors/disease	
Restoration of normality	*Acute infections/physio deficiencies*
Close approach to normality	*Asthma/dyspepsia*
Substantial amelioration with continuing disability	*MI, diabetes, lymphoma*
Symptomatic relief with residual major disabilities	*RA, schizophrenia, heart failure*
Minor or trivial improvement	*Dementia, OA, stroke, many cancers*

Fig. 2.3 A disease approach to health improvement: categories of intervention.

are short-term. Its main disadvantage is the reduced sensitivity to the wider influences on health and it could, perhaps, be perceived by some as a monopoly by the medical profession.

The social-environmental approach (holistic model)

The approach is based on the concept that the roots of most ill-health are social and environmental. While some of the parameters within this model are easy to define (eg housing and health), many are not (eg income, pollution, stress, diet, relationship, workload). Also, many of the required interventions are complex and require political action and the wider involvement of society in order to achieve change. Outcomes are difficult to measure and are long term. This approach does not fit well with current medical practice and education.

The educational approach (behavioural model)

The educational approach is based on the concept that the main causes of ill health are due to the individual's behaviour. While most such 'behaviours' are identifiable, it is difficult to quantify the exact causal relationship between any given one and the illness in question. Intervention(s) must be personal and their success depends on the individual's motivation. Society can regulate to protect others (eg the banning of smoking in public places). Outcomes are medium- to long term but not all are measurable. This approach fits well with current medical practices and education.

A mixed approach

In practice, it is very difficult to be a 'purist'. Any one approach to improving healthcare is inevitably, in fact, a combination of approaches. The fundamental criterion, we believe, is the ability to quantify and measure the process and its outcome.

Health Improvement Programmes (HImPs)

From the three health improvement models described above, we can conclude that to improve people's health it is important to consider *all influences that affect human behaviours and daily living*. Health Improvement Programmes (HImPs), therefore, are not about a narrow approach, a monopoly process, staying the same, doing our own things, or avoiding difficult issues.

HImPs should be *action-focused* through:

- Acknowledging the problem and its many dimensions, and doing things differently while building on current achievements
- Working together in full partnership and avoiding selection of the few
- Understanding and being sensitive to different perspectives.

Learning from lessons of the past and achieving such action-focused programmes are not simple given the current organizational culture of the public sector. Limited success or failures in the past can, in fact, be attributed to the rigidity of the organizational boundaries, the non-integration of action plans, and the lack of interest and involvement of agencies outside health. Above all, they can be put down to the fact that individual and public roles were never clearly specified.

The targets

HImP targets should be specific and measurable. They should address the most important health needs of the population and their wider determinants. The targets can be *population-wide* (for example, reducing the burden of coronary heart disease, pollution and chronic respiratory disease), specific to *high-risk groups* (for example, diabetic patients, young people and substance misuse), designed to meet the needs of the *individual* (for example, access to services, care pathways for severe mental disorder encompassing health, social, housing and other services), or a *mixture* of all three.

Addressing fewer targets and focusing on the most important pressing health issues, over the three-year (rolling) programmes, is a much better approach than attempting to tackle a long list of non-attainable targets. All targets should unite the NHS and its partners in achieving the ultimate objective of health improvement. Realism and pragmatism should be the guiding principles in any process of HImP development and implementation.

The process

If HImPs are to succeed, the processes of *development, implementation and measurement of the achievements* of these programmes must be clear. The role of each partner/participant must be specified and the magnitude of their contribution (management capacity, financial resources) specified.

HImPs should be developed at *three* levels:

1. Global or comprehensive: At this level, the lead agency (usually the health authority) will provide a general statement on the population health status, based on health needs assessments. Such a statement will identify, explicitly, how healthy the population is, the burden of various diseases (acute and chronic), the major determinants of health by diseases and client groups (women, children, young people, older people, minority groups, etc), and the availability of and problems with current services
2. Priority identification: Working with partners (local authorities, social services, education, police, health organizations [trusts, primary care groups], the voluntary sector and the public) to identify and agree the key priorities and areas in which health improvement is possible and how to address it locally. The identification of current and future resources (resource mapping), not only within health organizations but all possible health partners, should be part of the process at this level
3. Priority selection: Selection (from the above list) of a few (maximum 10, preferably less) issues to tackle jointly during the programme's life-span. Achieving a balance between national and local priorities is difficult in this respect. To ensure 'local ownership', a larger share should probably be given to local priorities. Each of these issues/areas should be the subject of a detailed *Sub-HImP*, which should, in turn, cover (in detail):

- the needs assessment of the condition in question
- the wider determinants and the contributing risk factors
- the current scientific evidence of the available interventions (health, social, economic, political)
- the current services available (quantity, quality, gaps, perceptions, level of satisfaction, etc) and current initiatives in progress
- the magnitude of the changes required to achieve improvements (need to specify measurable targets)
- the measures/interventions required to achieve the improvements
- the costs (and the opportunity costs of doing nothing)
- the specific roles and contributions of each partner
- the process and outcome (changes in health status, reduction in inequality, changes in service, level of satisfaction)
- a performance measurement framework (ongoing evaluation, feedback, public involvement and reporting).

The HImP document that results—published jointly with partners for consultation and subsequently for implementation—should be clear, use simple language (all jargon avoided or explained) and publically available. Leaders for each issue and named contacts for each action point should be specified. If HImPs are to work, the partners must be able to commit (and pool) their resources to the relevant activities. Some such activities, eg addressing wider health determinants, will be beyond their organizational boundaries.

The public's (and not just the relevant service users') involvement and support is very important to the success of HImP.

Measuring achievements

HImP is about achieving measurable improvements in health. Such measurement is not easy and, possibly one of the most difficult steps in the development of these programmes is the identification of specific measurements of process and outcome. Measurement could be high-level (health authority), geographical (borough, PCG, practice), condition/disease-specific, or client/group-specific. Linking HImPs to clinical governance will not only allow measurement at the grass root level and specific to individuals, but also greater commitment on the part of practitioners to their implementation (see appendix 1)[(20)].

Measurement of achievements could be categorised as follows:

1. Changes in health status, both general and disease-specific (high-level)
   - changes in mortality
   - changes in morbidity
   - changes in risk and contributing factors
   - changes in deprivation index
   - changes in peoples' perceptions of their health status
   - other social and economic indicators (employment, housing, income, etc)
2. Reduction of inequality—this could relate to geography, social class, or population subgroups, eg ethnic minorities

3. Target-specific measurements—these should be quantified and measured over a period of time and recorded as percentage change from baseline (eg percentage reduction in smoking among young people over three years)
4. Service-specific measurements—these include access, appropriateness, quality, outcomes and levels of satisfaction
5. Cost-efficacy measurements—of both the programme(s) and the intervention(s)—and the opportunity costs.

Conclusions

HImPs are the driving agenda for health policy in the UK. Through them, we are expected to address the wider determinants of health, improve the quality of and access to current services, and tackle health inequalities through a real partnership between health and partner agencies at the local level. There are many possible routes to improved public healthcare, but none could be described as simple or easy to follow. Whichever is chosen, if it is to succeed in improving the population's health measurably, there must be a clear vision, strong leadership, widespread determination and commitment (of resources, organizations and individuals), good planning, public involvement, and explicit means of measuring achievements. Additionally, local HImPs should be able to strike the balance between national and local priorities. If these requirements are addressed, HImPs have the potential to become effective models for improving healthcare in many countries, developing as well as developed.

Key messages

- There are many lessons to be learned from the past in guiding the development and implementation of HImPs and in monitoring their achievements
- Currently, the least acceptable 'face of the NHS' is the variation in clinical standards and practices within it
- There are many approaches to health improvement: for example, disease-burden, socio-environmental and educational
- If we are to improve health, we must consider all influences on human behaviour and daily living
- All HImPs should be clear in purpose, have measurable objectives, specify the role of each partner, and fully involve the public
- This UK model could be an effective means of health improvement in all countries of the world, developed and developing.

References

1 Newdick C. *Who should we treat?* Oxford: Clarendon Press, 1995.
2 Holland WW, Stewart S. *Public Health: the vision and the challenge*. London: Nuffield Trust, 1998.
3 *Royal Commission on the National Health Service*. London: HMSO, 1979 (Cmnd 7615).
4 *Committee of Inquiry into the Costs of the National Health Service*. London: HMSO, 1956 (Cmnd 9663).
5 Secretary of State for Health. *The Health of the Nation*. London: HMSO, 1992.
6 Department of Health. *The Health of the Nation—a policy assessed*. London: The Stationery Office, 1998. (HSC 1998/164).

7 Secretary of State for Health. *The New NHS: modern and dependable*. London: The Stationery Office, 1997.
8 Secretary of State for Health. *Our Healthier Nation: a contract for health*. A consultative paper. London: The Stationery Office, 1998.
9 Secretary of State for Health. *Saving Lives: Our Healthier Nation*. London: The Stationery Office, July 1999.
10 Rawaf S, Bahl V. *Assessing Health Needs*. London: Royal College of Physicians, 1998.
11 Helman CG. *Culture health and illness*, 3rd edn. Oxford: Butterworth-Heinemann, 1994.
12 Marmot M (Ed). *Social determinants of health*. Oxford: Oxford University Press, 1998.
13 Department of Health. *Variations in Health: what can the Department of Health and the NHS do?*. London: DoH, 1995.
14 Acheson D (Chairman). *Independent inquiry into inequalities in health*. London: The Stationery Office, 1998.
15 Judge K, Mays N. Allocating resources for health and social care in England. *Br Med J* 1994; **308**: 1363–6.
16 Department of Health, Welsh Office. *A policy framework for commissioning cancer services* (Calman-Hine Report). London: DoH, 1995.
17 Marinker M, Peckham M. Clinical futures: are as important to health policy as economic and social factors. *Br Med J* 1998; **317**: 1542.
18 Department of Health. *The National Health Service and Community Care Act 1990*. London: HMSO, 1990.
19 Rawaf A. *Managing change in the NHS*. MSc in Management dissertation. Bath: Bath University, 1997.
20 NHS Executive. *The New NHS: modern and dependable. A national framework for assessing performance*. Leeds: NHSE, 1998.

▶3

Healthcare needs assessment and health improvement programmes

Professor Andrew Stevens
Professor of Public Health and Head of Department, Department of Public Health, The University of Birmingham, Birmingham, UK

Dr Graham Bickler
Director of Public Health, East Sussex, Brighton and Hove Health Authority, UK

This paper reassesses the current approach to healthcare needs assessment in the light of the white paper *The New NHS: Modern and Dependable*[1] in which a wider constituency is given an interest in health needs through health improvement programmes (HImPs).

Healthcare needs assessment has always been necessary in any form of health service planning but in the early 1990s, under the previous government's health service reforms, it took on a more central role. The 1997 change in government with its emphasis on partnership continues to put healthcare needs assessment centre-stage, but with a more collaborative emphasis.

Stevens and Gabbay[2] identified four overlapping periods of changing perspective on need:

- social concern in the 1960s—identifying gaps in health service provision relating to deprivation and 'patchy' facilities
- rational planning in the 1970s—attempting to plan services systematically, but with no formal needs focus
- the resource allocation working party review in the 1980s—a focus on spatial inequity recognizing relative underprovision of services in different regions. Need was recognized and measured by surrogate means, notably mortality data
- the NHS review in the 1990s—needs identified by a variety of means (see below) such that services can be specified according to needs.

A fifth era of needs assessment can perhaps now be added:

- collaborative action in the 2000s—need for healthcare and other interventions to improve health collectively identified by health authorities and primary care groups (PCGs) and by local government, perhaps implying a careful selection of priority topics.

Objectives for needs assessment

Needs assessment has a variety of objectives:

- most enduringly from a health and local authority viewpoint, needs assessment is directed at the specification of health (and related) care services to be delivered

- to inform spatial allocation of resources between and within health authorities and also to inform social allocation between different groups
- a form of needs assessment is necessary to assess target efficiency (related to audit), ie do those who get a service need it and do those who need it get it?
- to generate a sense of involvement and ownership of the needs and service specification process.

While the central theme in the 1980s was the second of these objectives, ie the spatial allocation component, and in the 1990s it was the first objective, we are now moving to a period when social equity (a new part of the second objective) and corporate involvement (fourth objective) are moving nearer centre stage.

Definition of need

Almost irrespective of the objectives of needs assessment, the accepted definition of the need for healthcare is: 'the individual's or population's ability to benefit from health and related care'. Where there is no possible benefit, as is the case for all interventions which do more harm than good (eg the routine use of antiarrhythmics following myocardial infarction), it is difficult to argue there is a need. Provided 'benefit' is interpreted widely to include general wellbeing and benefit to third parties, the definition stands even where social equity is a principal objective.

The essential components of the assessment of the ability to benefit from healthcare are:

- incidence and prevalence, ie how many potential beneficiaries are there from an intervention or service?
- how effective are those services?

The assessment of need is ideally kept quite distinct from the assessment of demand (what people ask for) and supply (what is provided), although the three overlap[3]. A reasonable objective of health policy is to maximize the area of overlap of need, demand and supply by adjusting any of the three. The adjustment of supply is the obvious function of health service planning, but management of demand, and even modification of need by stimulating research on where benefit lies, are also important.

Approaches to needs assessment

While most approaches to needs assessment acknowledge, albeit tacitly, the 'ability to benefit' as the central feature of need, they often vary in other ways:

- Is the needs assessment about populations or individuals?—the methods of needs assessment for the two are not all that different. Individual needs assessment is sometimes the basis of population needs assessment where it is not prohibitively costly and inefficient to assess need in this way, ie where the caseload is small, cost per patient high, number of hidden patients relatively few or case-mix variability is high (eg assessing the needs of liver transplant patients or mentally disordered offenders)
- Is there a clear context for allocating scarce resources? Assessing need in the absence of any kind of resource framework often amounts to advocacy. The value

of needs assessment in the absence of any resource constraint or acknowledgement of other calls on resources is likely to be limited
- Is the needs assessment exploratory or definitive? Surveys exploring general health do not as their prime objective set out to establish needs from the point of view of service planning. However, they are a useful first step in providing an overview of equity and overall priorities
- Is the determination of the most important needs expert or participatory? Opinion is a frequent component of needs assessment and both experts and community participants have a role. The relative importance of each depends on whether the main goal is to be rational or to gain collective ownership.

Taking these considerations together, the classic population healthcare needs assessment:

- is population-based
- has a clear view of resource scarcity
- is definitive in its objectives
- principally uses expert (especially evidence-based) information sources.

There are three classic practical approaches to healthcare needs assessment which maintain these four features.

Comparative approach

This contrasts services received by the population in one area (or received by one group) with those elsewhere (or by another group). If nothing else is known about the optimal service to be provided, there is at least room for investigation if a local service differs markedly from those provided elsewhere. Comparisons tend to be powerful tools for investigating health services and have a wide currency in the growing 'variations literature'.

Corporate approach

This is based on assessing the alternative perspectives of interested parties including professional, political and public views. While such an approach can blur the difference between need and demand, and between science and vested interest, if undertaken systematically it gives rapid insights into major need—supply discrepancies and obtains detail on local circumstances. In short, the local corporate knowledge-base can be a valuable source of crucial information which it would be unwise to ignore.

Epidemiological/health economics approach

This approach addresses the definition of need as the population's ability to benefit by seeking information on incidence, prevalence and effectiveness (and cost-effectiveness) of services. As a general rule, and the foundation of the evidence-based medicine movement, a first priority is to establish the effectiveness of services rather than the number of those who might need them—in those cases in which services do not already have an established effectiveness profile, that is.

The new context

Health improvement programmes (HImPs) make the need for selectivity clear. In this context, a particularly useful perspective of healthcare needs assessment is to see it as centred on identifying and working on key priorities. Hooper and Longworth[4] suggest the following process:

- identify important health problems by systematically reviewing relevant information about a defined population
- use explicit criteria to choose the priority problems
- improve the health of people with each priority problem through developing a clear, systematic understanding of what the problem really is and working to improve it.

This can be thought of as adding detail to the fifth era of needs assessment (see page 23).

A wider range of stakeholders in the new environment underscores the value of this perspective. The NHS has been changed by the white paper: *The New NHS: Modern and Dependable*[1] and the public health paper *Saving Lives: Our Healthier Nation*[5] and, with respect to assessment, two issues need to be considered.

Breadth

Both the type of organization involved in needs assessment and the types of interventions that can be offered are broader. In the 1990s, health needs assessment considered services provided by NHS trusts and, to a lesser extent, general practices. It will now need to give a greater emphasis to the voluntary sector, local authorities and all NHS organizations (health authorities, specialist hospital providers, general hospital trusts, community trusts, PCGs and primary care trusts). As regards the types of interventions, the Government's emphasis on the wider determinants of health and decreasing health inequalities makes it clear that the concern is not just with health service interventions. Many activities undertaken by the voluntary sector and local authorities also affect health. For many public health practitioners, these elements of breadth are not new; but the new emphasis on 'joined-up problems' and 'joined-up solutions', demonstrated, for example, by the activities and interests of the Social Exclusion Unit, means that thinking like this will have to extend to all those in the NHS and not simply include public health practitioners who have always done it.

Securing agreement

The major cultural change in the NHS is the shift from a competitive culture to a collaborative one. Indeed, local authorities and all NHS organizations will have a duty of partnership placed upon them by the Secretary of State. While many believe that this is the right way to move forwards, it would be naïve to believe that this will be easy. Collaboration cannot be easily forced onto organizations and even with willing participants, a great deal of negotiation and discussion is required to reach agreement when interests do not coincide. Nonetheless, within HImPs it will be necessary both to agree what the priorities are and how each should be handled.

When it comes to setting priorities, this general scan of needs is required to allow appropriate focus. Broadly, priorities have to be negotiated, but the main consideration is an obvious gap between need and provision. High-profile issues have the attraction of highlighting the needs assessment process, but within each priority, needs assessment will determine what interventions improve health and the relative cost-effectiveness of each. The challenge is to draw on the best information and skills from all stakeholders so as to allow the process of needs assessment to be 'joined up'.

Entry points

One way of looking at how information from each sector can be analysed using the practical approaches to needs assessment set out above, is illustrated in Figure 3.1. This template demonstrates the approaches to needs assessment most appropriate for each sector.

In the hospital/secondary care sector, issues of effectiveness have been the most important entry into needs assessment. This is because of the development of the culture of 'evidence-based medicine' and because relevant information on what local services consist of is often available. In primary care, however, most of the descriptions of practice-based needs assessments[6,7] have used demographic descriptions of practice populations to illustrate differences between practices and have drawn on the experiences of primary care teams.

SECTOR / PRACTICAL APPROACH	Secondary care	PCG	GP practice	Local authority	
				Social services	Planning, leisure, transport housing, etc
How much?			Population register		Demography
Epidemiological					
What works?	Effectiveness issues	Key primary care interventions		Appropriate ?	Appropriate ? Effectiveness
Corporate		PCG board perceptions Systematic assessment of views across practices	Experiences of primary care teams	Political dimension, ie views of elected members	
Comparative		Interpractice variations			

Fig. 3.1 Contributions of the different sectors to three approaches to needs assessment.

In PCGs there is significant scope for a range of approaches to needs assessment and this could make them important contributors to needs assessment. For example, PCGs could and should be interested in whether or not key primary care-based interventions which have been shown to be effective are actually used (the epidemiological approach). Members of PCG boards are mainly clinicians, so their perceptions of need will be valuable (the corporate approach). It will also be interesting systematically to compare perceptions between practices and to look at inter-practice variations (see Figures 2.1 and 2.2 on pages 14 and 15).

For local authorities, the situation is a little different. In social services many of (what can be considered to be) the epidemiological approaches have been based on appropriateness, eg debates between residential and home care; skill mix and the boundary between health and social services. However, corporate needs assessment takes on a different dimension because of the rôle of elected local authority members. In effect, the corporate dimension is a local political one, but there are also many important effectiveness issues for local authority members They will need to consider which approaches actually work, eg How can exercise be increased in the population? How can housing design lead to increased social cohesion? What kinds of traffic calming measures decrease road traffic accidents?

These differences and similarities between the different sectors suggest an enrichment of the process. However, it does not need to lose its overall anchor of a population base, a clear view of resource scarcity, definitive service objectives and the use of expert information sources, with the exception of a more open approach to expertise given the nature of local democracy in local authorities.

Choosing priorities

This is an important process and must be influenced by national priorities, in particular the four *Saving Lives: Our Healthier Nation* priorities[(5)]. However, local priorities are also important and considerations of achievability, potential benefit and impact on inequalities should be central. Since many stakeholders will need to agree their priorities, an early agreement on the criteria for choosing them should make the process more transparent and easier.

Accidents among school children

Once a priority area has been chosen it is worth exploring how the knowledge-base can be assembled with the broader perspectives in mind.

Accidents are a national priority in *Saving Lives: Our Healthier Nation*[(5)]. Around 75 % of all deaths due to accidents are avoidable, the changing national pattern of accidents demonstrates that prevention can work and social class gradients have widened over the past decade. This is the type of issue in which interventions other than health sector interventions are likely to be important[(8)].

If we focus on school children, for whom many such accidents are road traffic accidents (RTAs), it is clear that each stakeholder has a different contribution to make. In the hospital sector the most important issue concerns the effectiveness of treatment: How are A&E departments organized? Are evidence-based interventions in place appropriately? Should regional trauma centres be developed? These are important questions in relation to need and, if dealt with properly, could reduce morbidity and mortality from accidents. As regards PCGs, while they may have a role in prevention via education, perhaps their most important contribution to needs assessment is promoting an understanding of the scale of the problem. To date, most of the information on accidents has been drawn from hospital databases. Primary care databases could contain much broader and richer information, but this would then need to be harnessed. A focus on accidents among school children could use primary care data to understand the scale of the problem.

Local authorities know a lot about where accidents (particularly RTAs) occur—but they are also concerned with the effectiveness of initiatives such as traffic calming measures, cycle routes, improving public transport and school-based education initiatives.

In the context of a HImP, this breadth and depth of understanding of a priority area can increase the range of interventions considered by a needs assessment exercise without jeopardizing the systematic approach. While the situation is different in other conditions such as childhood asthma—in which effectiveness in primary care is critical—this example illustrates how different approaches to needs assessment might improve the population's health overall.

Barriers to progress

Despite the potential, it is important to recognize that there are real difficulties.

Partnership fatigue

One of the effects of 'joined-up' thinking is that many individuals and organizations (eg drug action teams, responsible authorities groups, youth offending teams, regeneration partnership boards, joint consultative committees and others) are involved in multiple partnerships. Unless practical ways are found to focus on particular partnerships the process could become overwhelmed by a mountain of bureaucracy.

Data quality and compatibility

Many in the NHS are aware of the shortcomings of health data. In relation to public health, the wrong data are often collected and data are often of poor quality. Drawing on data from other sectors—particularly the local authority and primary care—offers opportunities but unless handled properly could simply produce more of the same. The NHS Information Strategy[(9)] may help, but information from outside the NHS should be looked at as critically as that from within the NHS.

Cultural differences

Many commentators have described how the words 'needs assessment' mean different things to different people in different organizations[(2)]. This is not just a technical issue, because it reflects the fact that different sectors and different professions approach problems from different angles. This is compounded by a historically different approach between sectors to the nature of evidence and the presence of an explicit local political dimension within local authorities. Solving this will not be easy, but an important starting point is to recognize it.

Other factors which are particularly relevant to PCGs include effective team working and the commitment of individuals to the process.

Conclusions

There are some clear messages about needs assessment in relation to HImPs, which draw on existing approaches but reflect a new perspective.

- It is possible to assemble the knowledge-base. In the new world this means being explicit and systematic, just as in the old world, but with greater possibilities for increasing breadth and the range of partners involved—perhaps being explicit and systematic is now even more important.
- It is important to choose real priorities. Such choices should be influenced by the potential benefit that can be achieved with any one of them, how achievable they are (both in political and technical terms) and the national priorities, eg those laid out in *Saving Lives: Our Healthier Nation*.
- Assessing needs is not that difficult. No matter how complex the theory and the technical and political difficulties, at its simplest, needs assessment for HImPs is about working with relevant stakeholders systematically and explicitly to identify important health problems and to use this information to improve the population's health. It might be that in a world of complex partnerships, hanging on to key messages and keeping things simple is the most important point.
- Needs assessment has the potential to confer great benefit. Not only does it offer a logical way of ensuring that priorities are directed at real health gain, but it also gives the needs assessors confidence in their understanding of the population's health and needs.

Key messages

- Healthcare need is defined as 'the individual's or population's ability to benefit' from health interventions and related care
- Healthcare needs assessment is an important first step in the development of any HImP programme
- Healthcare needs assessment can be undertaken in various ways, notably through 'corporate', 'comparative' and 'epidemiological' methods
- Needs assessment requires collaboration on setting priorities and acting on them
- Healthcare needs assessment will help to choose the real priorities that lead to wider potential benefits to individuals and population. Without proper assessment of needs, policies and decisions are taken in vacuum and will be less effective and not targeted.

References

1 Department of Health. *The new NHS: modern and dependable*. London: The Stationery Office, 1997.
2 Stevens A, Gabbay J. Needs assessment, needs assessment. *Health Trends* 1991; **23**: 20–3.
3 Stevens A, Raftery J, eds. *Healthcare needs assessment*. Oxford: Radcliffe, 1994.
4 Hooper J, Longworth P. *Health needs assessment in primary healthcare: a workbook for primary healthcare teams* (version 1). Leeds: NHS Executive, 1997.
5 Department of Health. *Saving Lives: Our healthier nation*. London: The Stationery Office, 1999.
6 University of York, Health Economics Consortium. *Health needs assessment step by step. A practical guide to practice based health needs assessment for GPs and primary healthcare teams*. London: Glaxo Wellcome 1997.
7 Shanks J, Kheraj S, Frish S. Better ways of assessing health needs in primary care [editorial]. *Br Med J* 1995; **310**: 480–1.
8 Roberts R, DiGuiseppi C, Ward H. Childhood injuries: extent of the problem, epidemiological trends and costs. *Injury Prevention* 1998; **4**(suppl): S10–S16.
9 NHS Executive. *Information for health: An information strategy for the modern NHS 1998–2005*. London: The Stationery Office, 1998.

▶4

Implementation: organizational commitment and stakeholders' involvement

Mrs Sue Gallagher
Chief Executive, Merton, Sutton and Wandsworth Health Authority, London, UK

Health defined in its broadest sense encompasses almost all activity—healthy living, healthy cities, healthy workplaces[(1)]. The health improvement programme (HImP) has excited us. Improving health and healthcare is a motivating objective: it matters to us as individuals, as family members, as employers, as employees and for society.

The conceptual framework of the HImP brings a number of challenging choices. Improving health and healthcare could include all the activity of the NHS, local authorities which focus on social and economic wellbeing and the independent and voluntary care sector. In practice, a HImP cannot cover all aspects of improvement work in these areas. To fulfil its purpose a HImP should:

- have a challenging, deliverable change agenda
- include all the key changes that are being planned for the next three years
- be meaningful to everyone who has a stake in it.

Dilemmas for health authorities

Figure 4.1 exposes some of the dilemmas for a health authority leading the development of a HImP. A cogent argument can be made for the end of each of the eight axes to be covered but what is the right balance?

The arguments surrounding some of these dilemmas can be illustrated as follows:

- There is strong support for a comprehensive context-setting direction statement including all the strategic changes, all the main themes of health improvement work and healthcare change priorities. Others say that while all this is relevant and will be happening locally, the HImP must be selective, meaningful to operational staff and to local people and specific about targets, milestones and tangible deliverables
- Each borough would prefer a HImP unique to it but many of the health improvement priorities and specific healthcare changes will be similar and duplication could be avoided by one document with borough-specific actions
- What vocabulary, presentation style and content will meet the critical appraisal of an informed member of the public who cares greatly but has no time for detail, *except* where it matters to him or his relative? What will show appropriate respect for the efforts of an expert who should be encouraged to continue to improve the care of patients with cancer or mental illness? Our context-setting discussion document on the HImP in Merton, Sutton and Wandsworth Health Authority, south-west London, stimulated 150 summarized pages of suggestions and comments on what needed to be included and the process for developing it. How with scarce resources can a response be provided that reflects this interest?

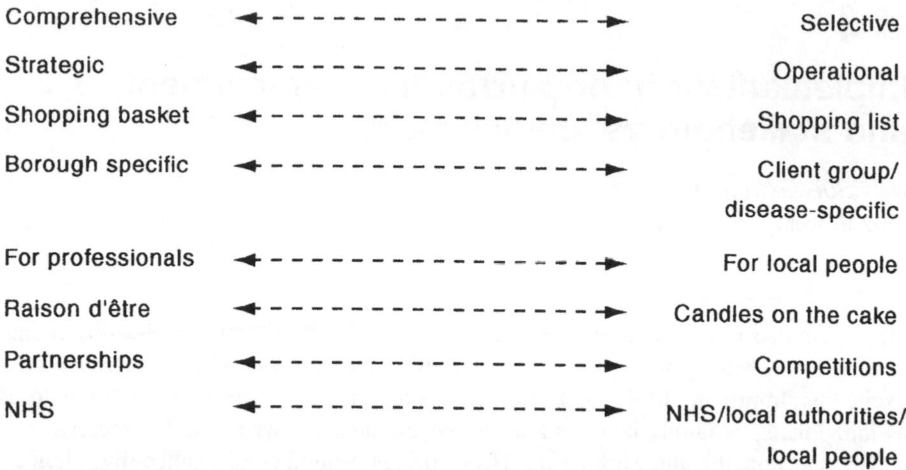

Fig. 4.1 What should a HImP be?

- How can it be ensured that the HImP continues to be the *raison d'être* of the local NHS and key partner agencies and does not descend into a birthday cake of sparkling candles, lit once a year and forgotten?

In this context, what do the duties and values of partnership and collaboration mean?

Duty of partnership with local authorities

Where there is one local authority/unitary council that matches the boundaries of the health authority, clarity of purpose and action is a practised art. Then there can be joint plans for community care, children, drug action, early years, crime and disorder, client groups, physical exercise, etc. Where there are three local authorities within the boundaries of one health authority, there will be three of each of these plans and a more complex construct for the HImP is necessary.

How can a HImP do more than just pay lip service to the endless hours of endeavour creating these plans and the detailed needs assessment and community profiling to establish the priorities within them? How is the work of other local authority departments that is critical to healthy environments—eg policies on pollution, food standards, transport, land use, regeneration, agenda 21 and education, much of which is also the subject of partnership working with the NHS and others—properly reflected?

Despite the frustration at 'another joint document', there is a strong drive from local authorities and the NHS to create one statement that acts as a comprehensive guide to all the key endeavours and tangible outcomes being worked on for the local community. Partnerships between statutory authorities are not, however, straightforward. Figure 4.2 illustrates some of the policy, political, financial, information and ownership debating points. These can cause great tension and require hours of negotiation behind closed doors and uncomfortable but pragmatic compromises.

Agreed priorities	BUT	?	Key priorities
Agreed investment plan	BUT	?	Unilateral action on £
One local needs assessment	BUT	?	Data gaps
		?	Systems incompatibility
		?	Withheld information
Delivery plan for national priorities	BUT	?	Local priorities
		?	Equal ownership
Joint action operational delivery	BUT	?	Politics
Agreed strategic direction	BUT	?	Members/local politics
		?	Decision-making processes

Fig. 4.2 Duty of partnership with local authorities.

Moreover, a duty of partnership may be meant to prevent unilateral action but human and political behaviour is not ultimately constrained by exhortations of partnership.

Is there space in anyone's stretched capacity to deliver the national priorities *and* some crucial different local priorities? Some of the priorities of the NHS may not be those of the local authority. In a world where demands and/or needs can greatly exceed readily realizable resources and where technology and skills shortages create opportunities and threats, decision making can be highly charged. Public legitimacy for change or local political support can be exceedingly difficult to achieve. What does 'agreed' plans mean in this context?

Duty of partnership in the NHS

Large acute hospitals may have 60 discrete specialties with a range of health problems presented to each. A large community health service or mental health trust may have over 20 discrete service programmes. A health authority may be host purchaser to six large trusts, have six primary care groups (PCGs), three local authorities and substantial purchasing power with many other organizations. Who should be engaged in the development of the HImP?

A dictionary of disease is massive. The possible healthcare interventions increase in double figures every five years. Causes of ill health can be summarized relatively easily but their manifestations cannot. A pragmatic approach with the HImP focusing on the main burdens of disease, main providers of care and main areas of service change may be realistic. However, this approach may disappoint many who are looking to the HImP to allow their focus of work to develop and to reflect their commitment to the wider health issues.

Three years in the NHS can encompass a massive range of change at a micro and macro level. If the HImP is to act as a statement of what will happen it should:

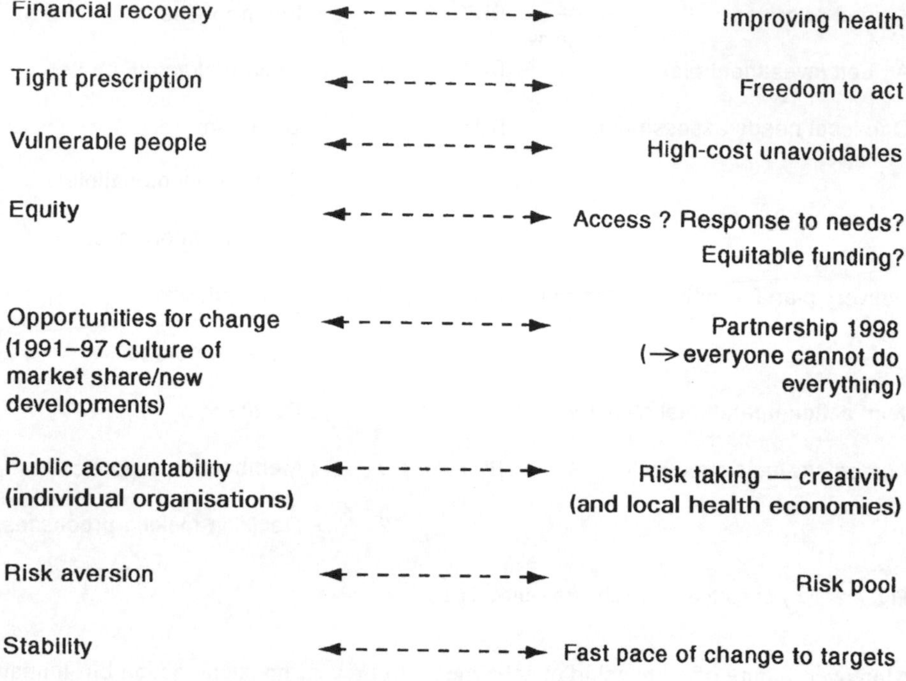

Fig. 4.3 Duty of partnership in the NHS.

- reflect the painstakingly negotiated large changes
- reflect the painfully determined disinvestments (to allow investment or to achieve or maintain financial balance)
- reflect the positively endorsed professional practice and health promotion changes
- reflect the prescribed nationally required changes
- anticipate where new technologies and new drugs may lead.

Public accountability means that it also needs to explain the rationale for difficult decisions such as those that require a balanced judgement between approaches that can be contradictory or pose conflicts and choices such as those shown in Figure 4.3.

Cultural change: from competition to collaboration

A massive cultural change from a competitive internal market to a collaborative partnership between organizations in the NHS should be reflected in the substance and process of the HImP. Similarly, general practice and PCGs should be engaged in its development and the value-base that promotes individual and organizational commitment to quality, equity, corporate behaviour and public accountability made explicit.

For many, a HImP would not be credible in this modern world without strong statements on clinical governance, recruitment and retention, information management & technology (IM&T), the achievement of accreditation or competencies and *Patient's Charter* priority areas.

The danger is that the HImP will become the dinosaur of the 1991 contract. It is a key public accountability document and there is a temptation nationally and locally to say 'it must be reflected in the HImP'. A brief paragraph may be appropriate, but too much about too many things and the HImP will become like the contracts: used by very few people, read by a few more and not user friendly to clinicians.

Key issues for delivering something that matters

The paragraphs above illustrate the complexity of taking the publicly acclaimed concept of the HImP into the practical reality of improvement-focused endeavour that is owned by many and summarized in a document.

The largest constraint for public services today, and for many other services, is the lack of time to do more. One of the major frustrations and fears is having to spread time so thinly that the quality of the outcomes and the process is compromised. A highly pragmatic and ruthless approach may have to be taken by the partner agencies managing the development of the HImP, under the leadership of the health authority, on how to address these complex issues. A balance is needed between the aspirations of the many stakeholders and what is workable and deliverable to achieve demonstrable benefits to the population.

Some of the key markers for success in developing a HImP that improves health and healthcare are:

- recognizing where to start
- critical mass of champions of change
- trusted relationships—shared values and aims
- cost-neutral, cost-saving or growth context?
- quick wins, longer-term staging posts
- major health problems/healthcare priorities/decisions
- realism regarding scarce time/capacity overload
- simple, relevant targets owned by professionals and meaningful to local people
- balance between government expectations and local realities
- action-based learning and organization and service-relevant action plans.

These, unashamedly, focus on endeavouring to make the HImP a meaningful, realistic, useful, outcome-driven process and product that has significance for the key people who must deliver it and who must remember it when difficult decisions are being taken in the community, hospital outpatient department or boardroom.

It is crucial that the jury does not sit on HImPs too soon; that a population focus drives the HImP and that the reality of complex change management, which needs to involve cultural and behavioural change, is recognized. A careful balance can be made between setting the strategic direction and ensuring operational implementation. The task is a complex one and lessons will need to be learned and shared. The creativity and vision is there, but developing the glue that makes the difference demonstrable for all to see will need much skill and hard endeavour.

Conclusions

The HImP is not only the masterpiece of the 1998 health reforms[1] but, more importantly, the cornerstone, in a legislative framework, of the new partnership agenda in and outside the NHS[1,2]. However, to achieve the massive changes necessary through real partnership, there must be realism and pragmatism in working together and a desire to collaborate and pool both resources and expertise to improve individuals' and populations' health. Such partnerships are neither dilemma-free nor straightforward. A balance, therefore, has to be struck between aspirations and what is workable and achievable.

Key messages

- The NHS is undergoing a massive cultural change from competitive market to collaborative partnership
- Partnership between statutory authorities is not straightforward
- A highly pragmatic and ruthless approach is needed in managing the development of the HImP
- The HImP should be a meaningful, realistic, useful, outcome-driven process and product that has significance for the key people who must deliver it
- The largest constraint for the public services today is the lack of time to do more
- A balance has to be struck between the aspirations of the many stakeholders and what is workable and deliverable to achieve demonstrable benefits to the population.

References

1 Secretary of State for Health. *The new NHS: modern and dependable*. London: The Stationery Office, 1997.

2 NHS Executive. *Health improvement programmes: Planning for better health and better healthcare*. Health Service Circular 1998/167. Leeds: NHSE, 1998.

▶5

Health improvement programme implementation: an example from general practice

Dr Geoff Roberts

Chairman, Surrey Heath Primary Care Group and General Practitioner, Camberley, Surrey, UK

While the term health improvement programme (HImP) is new[1], the activities required to deliver it are not. The new emphasis on 'joined-up' public health and the duty of partnership between health and social services provides an opportunity to build on and extend existing examples of good practice. The example described in this paper grew from one general practice's commitment to effective team working and has provided the focus for an application by an entire primary care group (PCG) to become a second-wave personal medical services (PMS) pilot[2].

Three recurrent themes have emerged from this work and they will come as no surprise to those involved in developing organizations:

- whatever you are aiming to achieve must feel important to all those involved
- the culture at the top of all relevant organizations needs to be supportive to enable implementation
- partnerships take time to develop and are highly dependent on the efforts of able individuals.

The lessons associated with these themes were learned along the journey from setting up an integrated nursing team through health and social needs profiling to the implementation of intermediate care services for vulnerable older people.

Capturing the opportunity

This opportunity arose when fundholding practices were given the responsibility for purchasing community nursing services[3]. The partners and practice manager decided to develop a management structure that would allow all the nurses to use and develop relevant skills regardless of their existing designated role. To achieve this a nurse co-ordinator was employed to manage the entire nursing team, including all practice and community nurses. Funding to evaluate this arrangement was sought and eventually secured from the nursing audit budget.

Two lessons were learned at this stage:

- if you hold the budget, people are very keen to please you
- never assume that you know what your staff want.

Although we consulted the nurses working in the practice, we did not allow sufficient time to explore adequately and listen to their concerns. We assumed that they would welcome the new arrangement and eventually they did, but there were some minor difficulties along the way.

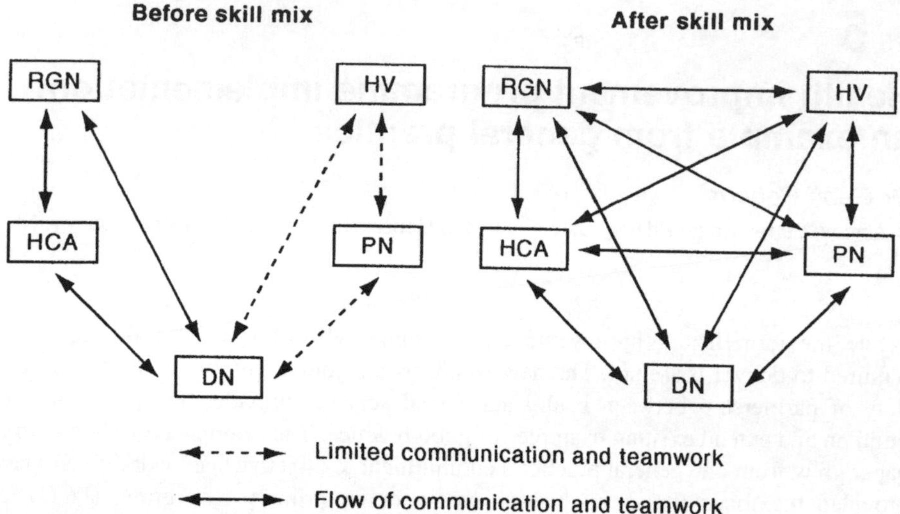

Fig. 5.1 Improvement in communication and teamwork with the development of a new management structure.
RGN = registered general nurse, HV = health visitor, PN = practice nurse, DN = district nurse, HCA = healthcare assistant.

The benefits are illustrated in Figure 5.1, which was produced by one of the district nurses at an evaluation meeting. The improvement in team working was brought about by improved communication, which, in turn, led to greater understanding of each individual's role. Communication is key. Perhaps, if the doctors and practice manager had communicated more effectively with the team initially, the introduction of the new structure would have been smoother.

Learning through experience

Find your own way

Managing the change provided a wide range of learning experiences. The changes associated with the nursing skill mix audit took place in a practice that had already developed a culture of change. From the first 'away day' in 1989, attended by 51 members (doctors, nurses and administrative staff) of the practice, little stood still for long. Even in this climate, it was noticeable how much anxiety was generated by the proposal of a single nurse co-ordinator to manage the skill-mix changes.

The first change required negotiation with the community unit, as it was then, about the new management arrangements. This was only possible once the practice held the budget to purchase community nursing services. Senior managers in the unit were facilitative, but some junior managers and team leaders were hostile. Regional support associated with the proposed skill-mix project helped to secure the right structure. A delay in securing funding to evaluate the project led to some time-marking once the nurse co-ordinator was in place, as it was felt to be important that no significant skill-mix changes should occur until the baseline audit was completed. After this, changes came thick and fast.

To understand how the changes were implemented, it is important to understand the management structure of the practice. There were five partners, one of whom was part-time, spending the remainder of his time in an educational role. The practice manager was fully involved in all partners' meetings and had an extended role, including that of fundholding manager. In the practice there were a whole range of multidisciplinary teams with particular clinical roles in: asthma, diabetes, child health surveillance, well woman activities, family planning, well person activities, etc. Each team now develops its own protocols and audits its own activities, which it reports to the partners at the regular Monday lunchtime clinical meeting. The partners hold an evening business meeting once a month.

Working with management consultants

While considering managing the change, we were approached by two management consultants who had secured regional funding to work in the area of health promotion. They saw their brief as enabling the practice to develop in whatever way it wished. They helped us to identify the problems of the present structure and to develop a practice forum which meets once a month with formal representatives of each group within the practice (two doctors, practice manager, nurse co-ordinator, health visitor, district nurse, practice nurse, midwife, administrative staff). There was some debate as to whether or not a member of the practice 'Patient Participation Group' should attend—so far, this hasn't happened. The function of this forum is to enable each group to raise new ideas or problems. It allows consultation with all groups before the implementation of any new ideas and has proved invaluable in debugging any impractical ideas.

In addition, the practice had an away day, which was attended by four partners, all community and practice nursing staff, the practice manager and two observers. This had been long awaited by the nursing staff as holding all the answers to their skill-mix question and one of the main outcomes was the identification of a multidisciplinary strategy group to take skill mix and other developments forward.

The partners met with the management consultants on two separate occasions to work through issues about how the partners related to each other and how the practice made and implemented decisions.

Implementation

At the end of this process, the management consultants met the strategy group, which consisted of two doctors, the practice manager, nurse co-ordinator, district nurse, health visitor, practice nurse and receptionist. These individuals were selected for their visionary powers and were different from those on the forum with the exception of the practice manager and nurse co-ordinator. It was agreed that the strategy group should attend a 48-hour residential workshop to take the skill-mix project forward.

Development of a practice profile

This process began in 1994 at a pleasant hotel on the south coast. On arrival, the strategy group defined its aim as 'the nursing team will use existing skills more effectively for the benefit of our patients and develop new skills as appropriate to the changing needs of the practice population'. The group worked together over two days, interrupted by some formal input. The main objective that emerged was to produce a practice profile involving all primary healthcare team disciplines and including mental health, social services, public health, housing and others as identified.

This was seen as the necessary first step in the effective targeting of nursing skills, as it was not possible to target these skills to the needs of our population until these needs had been identified. Social needs were included to provide a comprehensive picture because it was felt there is often a fine line between the need for nursing support and the need for social support. On our return, the nurse co-ordinator set about recruiting the other agencies through personal visits inviting them to attend an exploratory meeting. The participants included a GP, the nurse co-ordinator, practice nurses, district nurses, health visitors, a member of the practice patient participation group, practice manager, social services case managers, public health doctors (including the Acting Director of Public Health), an environmental health officer, a housing manager, a facilitator from the family health services authority (FHSA), a member of the community trust, a data analyst from the FHSA, the voluntary services co-ordinator, community midwives and five members of the local police force (including a superintendent).

This group rapidly established its mission—to develop a multiagency profile of the health and social needs of the people who live in the practice area in order to influence purchasing decisions. Specific objectives were also agreed:

- to expand and disseminate the existing *Directory of Community Organisations*
- where feasible, to make a comparison between practice data and geographical population data
- where possible, to make use of existing information
- where possible, to involve patients in identifying their needs
- to promote interagency working.

The immediate tasks were thought to be:

- to recruit other local practices to share data, thus developing a locality profile
- to bid for money from joint finance for an enlarged *Directory of Services*
- to collect data from all agencies and decide which are relevant.

The last task occupied the most time and provided the greatest learning insight. Information that existed outside the practice was usually based on geographical units of various kinds and for this reason it was decided that the area served by the practice should form our '*locality*'. Different agencies, not surprisingly, collect data in different ways, often using different geographical boundaries. Perhaps the greatest frustration was that data are often collected to manage budgets or inform some often ill-defined higher purpose within organizations and more useful information is either not collected or not held in a retrievable format.

The health and social needs profile was completed six months ahead of schedule due to the great enthusiasm of all involved. The findings included:

- practice turnover was 14% in the previous year (national average 9.5%)
- prevalence of asthma was higher than average

- A&E attendance rate was higher than average, particularly among young people, and was matched by a high admission rate.

From profile to specific recommendations

The profile has provided an excellent baseline and led to specific recommendations, including:

- the police should collect data on domestic violence and drugs on a geographical ward basis
- a multiagency data group should meet regularly to enable data to be gathered in the most efficient way
- to develop closer working with social services, a case manager should be attached to the practice on a sessional basis
- the practice should work closely with voluntary services to disseminate information about local organizations and services
- other practices should be encouraged to participate more actively.

Perhaps the most important outcome of this activity has been the development of an interested, committed, multiagency group which is keen to develop a more detailed picture of the needs of our community in order to influence the provision of services.

Hurdles to overcome

The greatest hurdle in the entire process was obtaining useful data about activity in primary care. Improving this lack of information is a major challenge for the new IM&T strategy[(4)].

The next major step was how to alter service provision. The project struggled a little at this stage. Although six practices had shared data, the project had emerged from and been driven by one practice: getting the others to buy in was time consuming. Eventually, an away day was organized to include representatives of all the practices as well as all other agencies. The King's Fund was engaged to facilitate, using the community-oriented primary care approach[(5)].

A few days before the event, the agreed funding was withdrawn, but due to an opportunistic social encounter with the Director of Public Health, immediately reinstated. Once more, support from the top of the organization proved invaluable. The away day took place at Woking Police Station, which proved a conducive environment. The group developed two clear priority groups—vulnerable older people and teenagers. It was agreed to concentrate on one and the former was chosen. The overwhelming feeling was that older people often end up in hospital inappropriately and the group wished to address this.

At this stage our police representative was promoted and that link was lost. Collaborative work is very dependent upon specific individuals.

Moving from a good idea to a change in service required detailed planning, training and dissemination. A smaller core group involving a GP, community nursing, social services and the health authority took the development forward. This group developed criteria (Table 5.1) and a protocol (Table 5.2) to enable patients to be admitted to a nursing home for up to two weeks.

Table 5.1 Criteria for admission to a nursing home

1. All patients must be Surrey Heath residents, registered with a participating practice and aged 65 years or over
2. Admission will be for a maximum of two weeks
3. Patient does NOT require hospital inpatient treatment
4. All patients will have identified nursing needs and an agreed nursing care plan signed by the district nurse (DN)
5. All patients will have a medical assessment/statement signed by the relevant GP
6. Patient and carer are willing to accept the plan
7. GP and DN team will provide cover to whichever home has the vacancy at the time
8. No patient will be considered for the scheme where there is a doubt regarding their ability to return home within the two-week period specified
9. Patients requiring psychogeriatrician input cannot be considered

A training day was organized to enable those involved in the system to comment on and adapt the processes. This was extremely well attended by both health and social services and led to detailed discussions on the joint assessment process. An addendum to the admission protocol was produced as a result of issues that emerged on this day (Table 5.3).

Piloting and evaluation

An evaluation group emerged to design a formal evaluation of the scheme and it was decided to pilot the scheme for a year. Perhaps due to it being summer, there was no

Table 5.2 Protocol for admission to a nursing home

1. All referrals to be directed through the designated GP and DN, medical and nursing assessment completed before contacting the co-ordinator and providing patient willing to accept scheme
2. Referrals can only be made between 9.00 am and 5.00 pm, Monday to Friday, excluding bank holidays
3. Co-ordinator to be contacted regarding availability
4. If bed not available, DN to complete referral/evaluation form and forward to co-ordinator for evaluation of unmet need
5. If patient accepted, DN to contact relevant nursing home and arrange admission and to inform co-ordinator accordingly
6. Co-ordinator to inform relevant care manager (community care manager [CM] for the area)
7. Contract to be signed within two working days of admission by CM, representative from the nursing home, patient or patient's representative. This will agree to purchase a bed for a minimum of one week and a maximum of two weeks
8. Transport could be provided with payment by negotiation
9. DN to complete nursing care plan and agree this with nursing home
10. Within one working day of admission, a discharge plan to be co-ordinated by the DN and the date and time of discharge arranged
11. One week from admission, discharge planning meeting to be held at nursing home with any of the following, as appropriate—patient, carer, nursing home representative, DN, GP, CM. Referral/evaluation summary form to be completed and sent with a copy of the nursing record sheet/care plan to the co-ordinator
12. Co-ordinator informed of discharge by DN. CM to be informed by the co-ordinator if not present at the discharge meeting

Table 5.3 Addendum to protocol for admission to nursing home

1. Geriatrician opinion may be needed; this could be accessed through the day hospital or by a domiciliary visit
2. Day hospital could also provide physiotherapy and occupational therapy service if deemed to be necessary
3. Community physiotherapy or community occupational therapy may need to be accessed through the GP
4. Specialist equipment to be organized by DN
5. DNs who have made a referral which has been turned down owing to no bed available should complete the paperwork as stated for evaluation purposes

funding available from the NHS. It looked, for a short time, as though the whole enterprise would flounder for lack of funding. However, the senior local social services manager on the group agreed to fund the pilot year from his budget—yet another example of the importance of senior support within the various organizations.

The scheme was successfully piloted and has been rolled out with 'winter pressures' money to cover the whole PCG area. Health and social services currently fund the scheme jointly. The collaborative spirit that developed has led to a joint application between the trust, social services and the PCG to become a PMS pilot to develop an integrated system of emergency care.

Barriers to change

The barriers to change lie with people and organizations. People are often threatened by change and are therefore resistant to it. This threat may relate to their incomplete understanding of the current system or the full implications of the change. Time spent exploring and explaining will pay dividends. On the other hand, the threat may relate to territorial issues or 'turf wars' which are harder to deal with. Another problem may be the loss of a key individual with a unique network and/or range of skills.

Organizational barriers often relate to funding systems. An example of this was encountered over transporting patients to nursing homes. The ambulance services had a contract to take patients to hospital (for admission) but no funds were available to take them to nursing homes. Reporting structures proved to be an issue as senior management figures came and went and less senior managers felt their position was being threatened.

Conclusions

Success breeds enthusiasm, but the financial priorities of the NHS have almost scuppered this activity on a number of occasions. This project led to a locality approach in an area where fundholding was the norm. This cooperative approach laid the foundation for the establishment of a successful PCG, which is developing rapidly into an effective organization. The emphasis on the health of the population and the configuration of services enabled a multidisciplinary group to develop its understanding of and skills in these issues. Our passage could have been smoothed and, if health in its broadest sense is to be a real priority, those striving to innovate within the system must receive consistent support.

Key messages

- While HImP is a new concept, the activities required to deliver it are not new to general practice
- Whatever you are aiming to achieve must feel important to all those involved
- Partnership takes time to develop and is highly dependent on the efforts of able individuals
- The process of practice profiling led to the development of an interested, committed, multiagency group familiar with the needs of its local population and able to influence the provision of services
- If health in its broadest sense is a real priority, those striving to innovate within the system must receive consistent support.

References

1 Department of Health. *The new NHS: modern and dependable.* London: The Stationery Office, 1997.
2 NHS Executive. *Personal medical service pilots.* Leeds: NHSE, 1997.
3 Department of Health. *Working for patients.* London: The Stationery Office, 1989.
4 NHS Executive. *Information for health.* Leeds: NHSE, 1998.
5 Gillam S, Plamping D, McClenham J *et al. Community-oriented primary care.* London: Kings Fund, 1994.

6

Becoming the future: changing clinical behaviour

Dr Anna Donald

Clinical Lecturer, School of Public Policy, University College London and Royal Free Medical Schools, London, UK

Professor Andrew Haines

Department of Public Health and Epidemiology, University College London and Royal Free Medical Schools, London, UK

As Michel Foucault described in *Birth of the Clinic*, 19th century healthcare was organized around political, social and technological conditions appropriate to the era[(1)]. Then, many people suffered from acute, infectious diseases and in the absence of clinical vigilance were likely to die quickly. Most patients were illiterate and deferent to authority and medical technology was still rudimentary, lacking safe anaesthesia or antibiotics. It was for the 19th century clinic that William Osler and Florence Nightingale prepared their students.

At the end of the 20th century, however, it is doubtful as to whether Osler's clinic remains the ideal model for healthcare provision. Both World Wars heralded major social and scientific developments that have irrevocably changed the way people live, get ill and die[(2)]. Even in developing countries, for example, most diseases are chronic and occur at home, the two most prevalent being heart disease and depression[(3)]. For rich countries, life expectancy at birth has more than doubled and the number living to 100 has more than quintupled. The cost and range of drugs and therapeutics has increased more than 10-fold; ageing 'baby boomers' are pushing Governments' limits on expenditure for health and social security; much of women's work is no longer free and time has become a precious commodity. Most people can read, write and participate in decisions about their own health and the cost of disseminating information has plummeted while the capacity to analyse it electronically has greatly increased.

New era and new type of doctor

Such changes have profoundly altered people's demand for healthcare and put pressure on clinicians to change their behaviour. For example, research repeatedly shows that people want more information about their conditions and have less time to wait to see health professionals. In Britain, the rate of law suits from dissatisfied patients continues to rise: official statistics show that the cost of meeting medical negligence claims rose from £80m in 1992–3 to £125m in 1994–5, prompting Lord Woolf's overhaul of medical negligence litigation[(4,5)].

While the 1970s saw broad recognition of the mismatch between 19th century ideals and 20th century conditions, resulting in initiatives such as WHO's Health-for-All-2000 programme, reform has been slow. Nearly 20 years later, although change is underway, most medical schools and postgraduate organizations still train and socialize doctors in Osler's image, in hospitals designed for a previous era, thereby creating doctors who lack some of the skills and much of the infrastructure to do what is required of them.

How then to proceed? What options are available to transform health services and the people that provide them?

Transformation of health services and practitioners

The first step perhaps is not to throw the baby out with the bath water. Although acute illnesses constitute a far lower proportion of cases than they did 100 or even 50 years ago, they still threaten lives and their management requires well honed skills and deep knowledge from health professionals. As a friend admitted recently, she might seek alternative therapy for back pain, but when acutely unwell with a kidney infection, she swiftly sought medical care. Doctors do not always get it right, of course, but that does not negate the fact that most people at some time during their lives still need diagnostic acumen and quick thinking during serious illness.

The second step is to decide what is needed to change clinicians' behaviour. There are two broad approaches.

Structural changes

The first approach involves altering the structures in which clinicians train and work (the International Monetary Fund approach). For example, it is difficult for clinicians to use research findings effectively if they cannot access computers, or to share and optimize working practices if hospitals and primary care units are forced to compete with one another for patients. Structural changes entail changing fundamental components of healthcare, such as its:

- methods of finance
- scale
- organizational structure
- accountability mechanisms (such as health improvement programmes) to stakeholders
- labour force skill mix and distribution
- training mechanisms
- means by which new technologies are developed and purchased
- integration with non-health sectors that have an impact upon health outcomes, eg environment, trade and industry.

In a democracy, structural changes can rarely be made by single players, but rather involve lengthy consensus-building processes, such as those leading up to the establishment of the NHS in 1948 and the transformation of the internal market structure into the more collaborative structures envisaged in the recent white paper, *The New NHS*[(6)]. Given current concerns about the cost of an ageing population and a diminishing workforce to pay for it[(7)], future structural changes likely over the next decade include substitution of doctors' labour by other health professionals; for example:

- nurse practitioners and nurse prescribing
- increased services and technologies for providing care in the home
- accountability mechanisms for medical decisions, such as routine data collection on performance indicators
- reduced medical autonomy around prescribing drugs and other expensive treatments.

Another likely development is a significant increase in user-friendly information available to the public about conditions and treatments, hence reducing the knowledge gap with health professionals.

Clinicians' behavioural changes

The second approach involves interventions that primarily aim to change clinicians' behaviour, which identifies the main obstacle to change as clinicians themselves, rather than the structures which create and maintain them. Typically, it entails the provision of incentives and disincentives and often involves:

- payment
- promotions (or demotions) in social status for certain activities
- requests and exhortations by influential bodies to change
- different kinds of educational interventions.

Examples in Britain include continuing medical education programmes to keep doctors up to date, 'fees for service' for certain 'desirable' procedures, such as screening for cervical cancer, and exhortations in policy documents to be 'clinically effective' when making clinical and purchasing decisions.

The 'behavioural change' approach is inherently more conservative than the 'structural change' approach, but is usually easier to introduce at a local level as it does not necessarily involve widespread consensus or major capital investment. Clinical governance and commissioning services to improve health through primary care groups (PCGs) are likely to motivate behavioural change in the future at primary and secondary care levels.

Behavioural shift

Which approach should be taken? The answer depends upon:

- diagnosis of the problem
- feasibility of alternative approaches
- timing of the change desired.

For any major transformation, both approaches are usually required, being somewhat interdependent. Structure influences the way in which people define themselves and people define themselves in a way that influences structure. For example, the creation of hospitals affects the way in which doctors perceive their roles and duties, while the way doctors perceive their roles and duties, in turn, affects the ways in which hospitals are built. So, for example, getting health professionals to consider reliable research findings when making clinical or purchasing decisions entails changing both the information-providing structures around them—libraries, computer terminals on wards, the structures which determine how research is produced and filtered—and clinicians' attitudes and skills in using research information, through interventions such as training workshops, public debate and financial or status incentives.

For successful change, some kind of behavioural shift, however achieved, is usually necessary before major structural change occurs, as successful structural change usually requires at least the implicit consent of many of those inevitably affected. Imposed structural change, without an 'incubation' period of attitude shifting, risks alienating people and making lasting change impossible. On the other hand, activities promoting behavioural change can rumble on for decades without lasting effect if they are not eventually made manifest in structures.

Implementing change

Which process?

Are some processes of change more effective than others? There are now many randomized controlled trials as well as several systematic reviews, based upon a literature of case studies and exploratory qualitative research, that suggest that some interventions work better than others at changing clinical behaviour across a variety of clinical settings[(8)]. These include:

- personal contact using outreach visits to alter prescribing habits
- manual or computerized reminders, eg to alter screening or prescribing behaviour
- multifaceted interventions that triangulate on an issue, rather than single interventions
- interactive educational meetings with peers to discuss ways to approach change.

Ineffective mechanisms include:

- distribution of educational materials without follow-up or discussion
- didactic educational meetings, such as lectures, rather than interactive ones.

Details of these trials, and new ones as they emerge, can be found in the *Cochrane Library*[(9)]. A 10-step checklist that we have found helpful in changing the way in which clinicians use research, and which draws from many of these ideas, is shown in Table 6.1[(10)].

In contrast, the 'evidence' for the efficacy of larger, structural interventions are rarely found in randomized controlled trials or other kinds of planned research, but rather in before-and-after routine data collection in individual health systems, cross-sectional comparisons between different health systems, such as those performed by the Organization for Economic Co-operation and Development, and descriptive case studies. While these evaluations often provide stark warnings against certain kinds of well intended interventions, accurate comparisons between countries and across time are often difficult to make, due to confounding factors that could not be controlled for, such as technological, cultural and demographic differences.

In Britain, it seems likely that future structural interventions, as well as more intimate, behavioural interventions, may be developed, evaluated and implemented using more formal methods. For example, new structural interventions, such as nurse

Table 6.1 10-step programme for changing behaviours and structures

1. Analyse in detail context in which clinicians work:
   - identify behaviour to change
   - identify levers, agents and rate-limiting steps at all relevant levels (incentives, enemies and allies)
   - consider grid of potential influencing (and overlapping) factors: social, emotional, financial, legal, physical, technological, professional
2. Involve critical mass of clinicians:
   - ownership/authorship of change, especially within isolated medical discourse/soliloquy
   - insight into what needs to be done
   - engagement with leaders *and* enough others to constitute critical mass
   - seeding if you have enough time
3. Communicate new model widely and coherently:
   - needs to make sense to people using it
   - people need to see where they are going
4. Select strategy and realistic time-frame:
   - eg collaboration, persuasion, attrition, seeding, confrontation, regulation, competition
5. Remove rate-limiting steps (RLS):
   - avoid demoralization
   - consider likely grid of RLS (social, emotional, financial, legal, physical, technological, professional)
6. Pick low hanging fruit and plan for short-term wins
7. Triangulate:
   - get model going with as many groups as possible (given resources)
   - address problem from different angles
8. Create accountability mechanisms
9. Create feedback loops, permitting (some) mistakes
10. Reward or punish
    - avoid demoralization

practitioners, could first be developed upon existing qualitative, exploratory research, and then assessed with a formal trial, before widespread implementation was adopted. It even seems possible that this evaluative, rather than ideological, approach to implementing structural change may extend to other areas, such as education and criminology. Members of the Cochrane Collaboration, for example, are currently searching for trials about educational interventions—changes in classroom size, teaching methods, payment methods for educational services—in order to find interventions to help our school system. One wonders what the NHS, national curriculum or prison services and rehabilitation might look like had previous governments adopted such an approach.

Processes and outcomes

Whatever the precise route chosen, attention to processes as well as outcomes seems to be as important to policy as they are to research. Just as one would not expect to evaluate reliably nor license a drug using a case-control study, it seems unrealistic to attempt to steer a cohort of practitioners towards some policy goal without paying attention to the processes one chooses to get there. The good news is that reliable information about the best uses of such processes seems likely to be available. Then, perhaps, creating a 21st century clinic capable of meeting the needs of the population may not seem so daunting.

Conclusions

With the explosion in information technology, easy access to information and increased public expectations and demands—both for information and health care, clinicians need to adapt to a new era of healthcare systems. Structural and behavioural changes could begin at medical school. Interventions are available to influence clinical decisions and practices.

Key messages

- People's demand for healthcare and patients' dissatisfaction have put considerable pressure on clinicians to change their clinical behaviours
- Changes are needed in both structures and behaviours
- Structural changes should start at medical school
- Behavioural changes can start with individual clinicians and do not necessarily involve widespread consensus or major capital investment
- Attention to processes of change as well as to outcomes is as important to policy as it is to research.

References

1 Foucault M. *The birth of the clinic. An archaeology of medical perception.* London: Tavistock Publications, 1973.
2 Hobsbawm E. *The age of extremes. A history of the world, 1914–1991.* New York: Pantheon, 1994.
3 Desjarlais R, Eisenberg L, Good B, Kleinman A. *World mental health. Problems and priorities in low-income countries.* Oxford: Oxford University Press, 1995.
4 Dyer C. Medical litigation faces British revolution. *Br Med J* 1996; **312**: 330.
5 Secretary of State for Health. *The new NHS: modern and dependable.* London: The Stationery Office, 1997.
6 World Bank. *Averting the old age crisis: policies to protect the old and promote growth.* Oxford: Oxford University Press, 1994.
7 Haines A, Donald A. *Getting research into practice.* London: BMJ Publications, 1998.
8 *The Cochrane Library.* Issue 4. Oxford: Updated Software, 1998.
9 Donald A. *Front line EBM project: final report.* London: North Thames Regional Office, R&D Programme, 1998.
10 Poullier, J. *OECD health systems: vol I—Facts and trends 1960–1991; vol II—The socio-economic environment and statistical references no 3.* Paris: OECD, 1993.

▶7

Local government and health improvement programmes

Mr Andrew Boatswain

Director of Solace Enterprises Ltd, Former Chief Executive,
Swansea City Council, UK

There is good news about the way local authorities perceive their role in relation to the changes in health and social services currently in progress. The performance of some councils, has, of course, been called into question—they have been called intransigent and unwilling to embrace new ways of working—but at least some of this criticism is unfair. The number of really poorly performing councils is declining but the extreme examples hit the headlines and impact disproportionately. My current role often involves talking to councils about recruiting a new chief executive. Almost without exception, councils approach this from the direction of bringing in someone to the post who will help them change—help them change more quickly, offer new ideas and modernize their approach.

Old image of local government

Chief executives do not leave every day and different councils move at quite different rates, so pace of change is far from uniform. Also, what one council may see as radical, another sees as 'old hat'. Generalizations are therefore difficult.

Sadly, one sometimes detects a patronizing tone in what is said about local government, especially in some of the words emanating from Whitehall. That is not to say that councils are not sometimes their own worst enemy—there are still pockets of underachievement, some poor public relations and some intransigence. It would be idle to pretend that things could not improve.

A perception held within local government is that much of the innovation within it is coming from the councils themselves and that the Government has seized on some of the best practices that already exist and is now promulgating these (sometimes as its own). It is now commonplace to accept that tackling some of the major issues in our society can no longer remain the responsibility of single organizations acting autonomously. While the history of successful collaborative activity across many policy areas is variable, it seems to some of us that it has been worse in government than anywhere else. Not so long ago, when I was working in Wales, we used to look with astonishment at some of the barriers different government departments erected between themselves. Attempts to deal with this in the last year or two have so far only touched the margins. The good news is that the Government shows awareness of these problems and is grappling with solutions.

Partnership: new attitudes, skills and structure

This is not to suppose that all is well with councils and other public sector agencies and that the government alone has got it wrong in the past. Working in partnership calls for new attitudes, new skills and new mechanisms or structures. We are at the start of a long road of discovery and it would be wrong to pretend that anyone knew all the answers. Many organizations are unnecessarily defensive and there is often a culture more concerned with erecting boundaries than working collaboratively. Few public servants are equipped with the skills to work in partnership and people need to be trained quickly if things are to change.

New duty to promote health

Against this background, however, local authorities will welcome a new duty to promote the health and wellbeing of their local population and it would be extremely surprising if there are currently any councils that do not recognize the absolute requirement to work in a range of partnerships to achieve this and their other community responsibilities. This does not, of course, mean that they are equipped to do it well. The point is that there is an understanding of the need to work differently from now on. The benefits of closer partnership between medical and social care versus the shifting of responsibility between the two are well documented.

It is also well recognized that most of the NHS must be feeling the impact of change upon change. Because the NHS is widely perceived to have a greater direct impact on the lives of everyone in society than many other public services, successive governments do not lack the incentive to make changes to it with, one supposes, the object of improving it. This continuous changing of organizations and structures can be distracting and, for some, demotivating and divisive. Successive governments at least appear to have a purpose and, although it seems to mean sharp changes before the last change has had a chance to become embedded, there is, one would suppose, a logic to what is proposed.

Barriers to partnership

Restructuring and organizational development

The problem is that central Government does not know what to do with local government and, in any case, there are few votes in whatever it does. The last so-called reorganization actually worsened the situation. The confusing mix of unitary and two-tier structures across England has no rhyme or reason and makes for more difficult partnerships. In Wales there are too many unitary councils, some of which are very small and desperately under-resourced.

Despite the mention above of the willingness of councils to embrace change, sometimes it is slow and hard-going for all concerned. Changes can be slow to take effect and some things seem to be forever enshrined in the culture. Thus, there are still many councils in which a Victorian councillor would feel at home—albeit unfamiliar with the topics of discussion. In fact, many local governments are still applying 19th-century structures to late-20th-century problems.

This situation is likely to change in the next couple of years because the Government is forcing the issue, but a change in structures alone will not solve some of the underlying ills in local government such as the reluctance of people to come forward as councillors (all parties struggle to find candidates), uncontested seats, shadow candidates being elected to their surprise and (sometimes) the dismay of others and the poor turn-out at elections generally (the lowest in Europe). Councillors are keen to point out their unique legitimacy as elected bodies but it is hard to sustain that when so few vote for them.

Power games

Some councils have a problem with councillors' reluctance to give up what they see as power or 'sovereignty'. This is, of course, critical to successful partnership since partnership by its very nature is about sharing and 'give and take'. This is a nettle that has to be grasped.

Local government finance

The Government's legislative plans for local government are, regrettably, only good in parts. The greatest 'fudge' comes with finance; there has been a deafening silence over anything touching the fundamentals of local government finance. The moves proposed on council tax capping and business rates are tokens only and reform of the latter appears to have been shelved indefinitely. There is a fundamental weakness in the way that councils are so significantly funded by central government rather than local sources. Unfortunately, better options like local income tax appear too risky to the Government after the failed introduction of the poll tax.

So the optimism in local government is tempered by disappointment that the Government has failed to be radical enough and that the new thinking is largely confined to political structures such as the concept of the directly elected mayor. New structures are beguiling to some but do not, in themselves, improve services and are unlikely to help significantly.

Councils have managed to cope with huge changes in systems, people and skills. Similarly, the most recent reorganizations were marked by huge upheavals which could have seriously disrupted services but did not. Local government has a good track record of coping with major changes. This is good news for all collaborative working arrangements. Increasingly, councils recognize the need to predict and plan things in partnership in a proactive rather than reactive way. At last we are moving away from crisis management.

Local government role in delivering the health agenda

Reference was made above to the likelihood that councils will see the role of the NHS as more important than most local government services. This is being realistic. However, there are many councils that have been saying for some time that problems of social exclusion need to be tackled at their roots. Most councils will probably have antipoverty strategies, community safety plans, environmental strategies, etc, in place. They may not always be integrated and even if some of these plans do not cross the boundaries of different agencies, their very existence means that councils are thinking about the impact of a wide range of services and actions on the lives of their citizens. The fact that health is seen as of such overriding importance to councils is itself a key to joint working between councils and the NHS.

There are some excellent examples of joint working and joint investment plans (JIPs) with social service departments to deliver integrated community care programmes. There is good practice involving all sorts of partnerships with health authorities, other public bodies, the private sector and voluntary agencies. It is almost invidious to mention specific examples, but there are several interesting examples from Somerset, my county. Much work has already been carried out in trying to consult widely on health improvement plans (HImPs). This demonstrates the willingness there is to work together, to give and take, to share problems and to try to find joint solutions. The new partnership boards forged by North Tyneside Council and the community and in the London borough of Havering are good examples of innovative ways of working with partners.

Somerset may not be the most progressive council. There are many other examples of good or best practice which need to be collated and disseminated so that everyone can benefit from looking at what has worked elsewhere and then choose and adapt the solution that fits local circumstances the best. Finding local solutions is critical.

Drivers for collaborative working

There are at least three main drivers for collaborative working.

Harnessing public opinion

The age of public consultation is with us. Some councils have tried to seek the views of the public for several years with mixed success. Now public consultation is fashionable and many councils are anxious to consult more widely and effectively but are uncertain of how to do this. They are concerned that they only reach those with interests to protect or those who shout the loudest. There is often apparent apathy from the public. More and more councils want to shift towards greater public involvement and prepare true community plans, but the results are still very ‘patchy’.

Public involvement is an area in which many health authorities have worked hard and have something to offer their council counterparts. Working together, the power of council and health authorities to involve communities should be compelling and might grab the interest of those whom councils have found it difficult to engage thus far. There are already good examples of joint working on consultation. Joint working will be essential to the preparation of HImPs and will more than double the impact of consultation.

Finance

All public services are short of cash. To make health improvement a reality, health authorities must lead alliances that demonstrably stretch resources further. This requires compromises, especially the willingness to review all priorities. Despite the difficult resource decisions some councils have to take, one can assert with confidence that every local authority can find money for some political priorities if it really wants to. The trick is to find where priorities match and to make a real impact in these areas by joint funding. There are clear indications that the Government will use its powers of direction here by increasingly linking resources of joint bids and programmes—JIPs and healthy living centres are examples of situations in which partnership working is essential to secure funding.

Outcomes

If councils, along with other partners, can see tangible benefits from an investment in partnerships, these benefits will be obvious to all. We need to build on successes. To do this, locally agreed targets that are measurable in the short and longer term are essential. Health authorities and primary care groups have to bind councils (and other partners) into the partnership arrangements by showing them the benefits in terms that match their interests and agenda. This will not always be easy because it takes time to both build up partnerships and to allow their benefits to become obvious. The message is that this is fertile ground.

Partnership: investment in people

The current emphasis on the importance of partnerships tends to revolve around structural and organizational imperatives, but the effectiveness of such ventures rests largely with the people involved with the process and their capacity to apply collaborative skills and a collaborative mindset to the task. The fashioning of relationships is a job for talented practitioners.

Councils almost without exception are rewriting the skills needed for their most senior posts to include the ability to work in partnership with other organisations. These skills are not always resident in local government officers, although there is a new generation of managers coming through that is not so imbued with professionalism that it is constantly seeking to defend boundaries.

There is, as yet, little interchange between managers in the NHS and local government. However, some council recruitment from the NHS into senior posts can be welcomed. These 'joint appointees' may be unusual but are certainly perceived as inspired. The wider knowledge and understanding now resident in these organizations will help to build bridges and, thus, stronger partnerships.

Positive steps need to be taken to allow managers in the public sector to acquire better collaborative skills. Secondments, exchanges, work shadowing and joint training initiatives should be developed if the opportunities are to be maximized and it is to be ensured that managers understand their collaborative capability. A friend of mine calls people who can work across organizational boundaries 'spanners'. I think more spanners are needed in the works.

Extra management resources

A worry, perhaps, is the time and staff resources necessary for partnership working. Senior managers are not only trying to cope with the internal changes of the 'modernization' agenda, but are also adding health, crime, drugs and other partnerships to their already heavy workload. Without proper extra resources and sensitive management to cover the partnership duties, the latter may become rapidly marginalized.

Conclusions

Despite negative perceptions, rigid structure and a lack of skill in collaborative work, local governments across the UK are changing and preparing, through structural and managerial changes, for the challenging agenda associated with HImPs[1] and the other elements of *The New NHS*[2]. Joint vision, pooling resources and expertise, and joint appointments of senior officers are some of the positive approaches for closer alignment between the organizations serving the local health economy with the joint objectives of identifying and meeting the health and social needs of the local population.

Key messages

- Different local authorities change at a different pace
- The history of collaborative activities across many policy areas is variable
- New partnerships require new attitudes, skills and structures
- With all the other pressures and time constraints on top-level managers in health and social services, HImPs will run the danger of being marginalized unless adequate senior staff resources are drafted in
- Local authorities welcome the new duty of promoting the health and wellbeing of their local population
- There are many barriers to full partnership which need to be overcome
- Innovative approaches are being made in developing joint vision, pooling resources and skills, and joint appointments
- Partnership is about 'give and take'.

References

1 NHS Executive. *Health improvement programmes: planning for better health and better healthcare.* Health Service Circular 1998/167. Leeds: NHSE, 1998.
2 Secretary of State for Health. *The new NHS: modern and dependable.* London: The Stationery Office, 1997.

▶8

Health improvement programmes and the public

Mr Gary Fereday
Association of Community Health Councils for England and Wales, London, UK

Current Government health policy stresses the need for increased collaboration between different agencies and emphasizes the importance of public health initiatives and the need for greater partnership between the professions and the wider public: 'Joined-up government' is the new buzzword around Whitehall. Health improvement programmes (HImPs)[1]—local strategies for improving health and healthcare, drawn up by health authorities in consultation with health professionals, local authorities, local businesses, patient groups and representatives of the wider community—embody these goals within the health service.

Democratic accountability of the NHS

As a public service funded from direct taxation, there is a clear case for democratic accountability in the NHS. Yet there are no directly elected representatives on NHS governing bodies and the service is, in effect, only accountable to the Secretary of State for Health. Community health councils (CHCs) are the only bodies that ensure a more direct level of accountability to local communities.

As statutory representatives of patients and the wider community, CHCs will play a key role in ensuring public participation in the HImP process. However, the extent to which HImPs will detail service provision is not entirely clear as the direct responsibility for commissioning of care will be largely devolved to primary care groups (PCGs)[2]. Hence, CHCs will need to develop a role in monitoring PCG commissioning to ensure that local community needs are met in the wider framework of the HImP.

Health improvement versus service delivery

CHCs have broadly welcomed the HImP concept. The refocusing of NHS thinking towards health improvement rather than service delivery should, in the longer term, bring much greater benefit to the health of the general public. The proposed reduction of health inequalities is particularly welcome after the Government-commissioned 'Acheson Report' recently concluded that: 'Although average mortality has fallen over the past 50 years, unacceptable inequalities in health persist. For many measures of health, inequalities have either remained the same or have widened in recent decades'[4].

However, this emphasis on health improvement, partnership working and public health measures will inevitably lead to resources being shifted to different priorities. The achievement of long-term national and local priorities (particularly the reduction in health inequalities) will, without additional funding, almost inevitably result in cuts to established services. Local communities must participate in such debates if the public is to maintain its support for the NHS.

Link between the NHS and the community

Mechanisms already exist for consultation—health authorities are required to consult CHCs when they are considering proposals for substantial changes to service provision[(5)]. While an essential safeguard, this will not be enough to ensure that HImPs comply with the need to ensure that all parties, including local communities, participate at all stages of the process. CHCs are uniquely placed to help ensure public participation in the process.

Operating with only a handful of paid staff (two or three full-time equivalents—often fewer in Wales) and with members offering their time for no remuneration, CHCs provide a low-cost health service 'watchdog'. While CHCs are not without some criticism[(6)], they have proved resilient and demonstrate that they can make a difference[(7)].

Founded in 1974 following a series of scandals involving long-stay hospitals, CHCs constitute a link between the NHS and the community they serve, separating the management of service provision from the representation of patient and the wider community interests. At the time of their creation, 'consumerism' was a rising force and the need to give voluntary groups a voice was acknowledged by allowing voluntary bodies to elect representatives. Also at that time, it was considered important that there was more local authority input into the NHS; hence local authority representatives also made up the membership of the newly created CHCs[(8)]. It could said that for 25 years CHCs have been 'joining up' the expertise of members of a range of bodies from the wider community.

Local people and HImPs

CHCs have broadly welcomed the Government's concern with the wider determinants of health, including the environment, housing conditions and levels of unemployment and poverty. The Association of Community Health Councils for England and Wales (ACHCEW) has previously highlighted the need for increased co-ordination between employers, local authorities, other agencies and the NHS[(9)] and argued that 'radical steps will be required to make significant progress in tackling avoidable ill-health in the foreseeable future'[(10)].

The HImP process may well offer health authorities the chance to take such steps. According to the Government's guidance, the aim of involvement and consultation in the HImP process is to ensure 'the widest possible local involvement from the outset, rather than consultation on a near-final product and local communities need to have a real opportunity to shape the HImP so they feel ownership of its objectives and are committed to its implementation'[(11)].

While such a commitment to public participation in the process has been welcomed by CHCs, there is no prescribed method of consultation or involvement.

Methods of consultation

There are many ways of involving and consulting the public and the literature available to health service managers is quite considerable. The issue is complex, the terminology is often confusing and there is a myriad of relationships between the different individuals and groups concerned. Given the enormous pressures that health service managers face in a tightly cash-limited service, some of them are unclear of the best way to proceed with public consultation.

Often the terms involvement and consultation are used interchangeably, leading to confusion as to how the public can participate in the healthcare debate. Public *consultation* should be seen as a process that seeks the views of a broad constituency of people and *involvement* as the inclusion of the public (often groups of users) in the planning and management of services.

The is a wide range of consultation methods including citizens' juries, focus groups, interviews, surveys and public meetings[(12)]. Some target patients, others the wider community. Some methods allow for informed discussion and debate, while others do not. Public involvement ranges from the involvement of the individual user in their own care through to the concept of community development, enabling communities to set and direct their own health agendas.

Given this range of methods there is a need for a body, independent of health service management, to monitor health authorities' consultation/involvement practices. This body must ensure that members of the public participate in the most appropriate way and that the health authority uses the information gained from the consultation/involvement in its decision making to help shape the HImP.

The CHC membership structure has the potential to enable these councils to bring a unique perspective to the consultation and involvement process with one-half of the membership selected by local authorities, one-third from the voluntary sector and the remainder appointed by the Secretary of State for Health or the Secretary of State for Wales (this may change with devolution of power to the Welsh Assembly). The CHCs' wide-ranging contact with local community groups reflects the partnership approach that embodies the HImP process.

CHCs will need to be involved from the outset of the HImP process. Indeed, the guidance states that 'each HImP should identify those areas that will be subject to detailed review for the next round and ensure that the timetable allows for in-depth involvement at a stage sufficiently early for partners genuinely to influence the structure and development of the plans'[(11)].

HImPs should not be processes that only consult and/or involve the public at periodic intervals: public participation should be an integral part of the process at all stages.

By not prescribing a particular method of public participation the guidance allows the adoption of methods that reflect the needs of the local community. It also allows health authorities to adopt methods that are unsuitable or methods designed simply to legitimate decisions that have already been taken. CHCs will need to develop their role in ensuring health authorities adopt the most appropriate means of consultation/involvement and that HImPs genuinely reflect the input of the community.

The guidance states that 'each HImP should record who has been involved and how'[(11)]. If the wider community input into the process is to be properly measured, then a record of how the community's views have affected decision-making is vital.

CHCs are aware that the process does not envisage formal consultation on the HImP itself; they will therefore need to become proactive in demonstrating the benefits of their involvement. However, the guidance is quite explicit that 'specific proposals for substantial service changes arising from the HImP would be subject to the existing consultation procedures'[(11)].

The 1996 CHC Regulations, which require health authorities to consult CHCs, will not be affected by the HImP process.

The guidance does identify particular groups that should be involved in the HImP process, stating that 'It will be particularly important to take positive moves to involve those groups (eg children, older people, black and minority ethnic groups) who are underrepresented or hard to reach through the NHS' traditional consultation methods and consultation partners'[(11)].

Key roles of the CHCs

CHCs have considerable experience in conducting research and advocating for improvements in services for children, older people and black and minority ethnic groups. Many have working groups or subcommittees that explicitly examine these areas of healthcare. Indeed, there are a number of key roles that CHCs are ideally placed to perform:

- Direct representation on any 'partnership council' or steering group that is set up involving the different partners to agree the HImP
- Advising the health authority on ways of ensuring public participation at all stages of the HImP process
- Scrutinizing the HImP document to ensure that the public has participated in the most appropriate way and that the findings of the involvement/consultation have genuinely been considered in the decision-making process.

HImPs 'should be published annually and made widely available in accessible forms (which may include public summaries and Braille copies)'[(11)]. Again, CHCs could play a role in ensuring that accessible forms are available and ascertaining whether or not they are reaching the required target audience.

CHCs and primary care groups

PCGs will play a central role in the HImP process, as they will become the main commissioning agency of services to deliver the HImP objectives. Each PCG board is required to have a lay member representing the interests of the wider community.

Again, there is an obvious role for CHCs who have both the expertise and the links with local communities to give help and advice to appointed lay members. Lay membership of bodies heavily dominated by professionals like the governing bodies of PCGs is daunting for even the most assertive individual. Any support the appointed lay members receive should help them effectively discharge their duties.

PCGs will have the power to co-opt additional members on to the board. These co-opted members will become associate members of the board but will not have a right to vote. Associate membership, as outlined in the guidance, offers CHCs the opportunity to gain the speaking observer status that their national association (Association of Community Health Councils for England and Wales [ACHCEW]) previously called for. Many PCGs have already seen the benefits of awarding such status to CHCs.

Conclusions

CHCs have the potential to play a unique role in assisting the Government in its drive for 'joined-up' government through the HImP process. With their membership drawn from the local voluntary sector and local authorities, CHCs are well placed to represent the public interest, while also contributing knowledge about the diverse range of agencies and bodies that will need to be involved in the HImP process.

Key messages

- Greater emphasis on the wider determinants of health (environment, housing, employment, wealth) is welcomed
- Greater partnership between the professions and the wider public is needed
- CHCs will play a key role in ensuring public participation in the HImP process
- As healthcare commissioning will be largely devolved to PCGs, CHCs should develop a clear role in monitoring PCGs
- All possible methods of public participation should be explored.

References

1 NHS Executive. *Health improvement programmes: planning better health and better healthcare.* Health Service Circular 1998/167. Leeds: NHSE, 1998.

2 NHS Executive. *The new NHS: modern and dependable: establishing primary care groups.* Health Service Circular 1998/065. Leeds: NHSE, 1998.

3 Secretary of State for Health. *The new NHS: modern and dependable.* London: The Stationery Office, 1997.

4 Acheson D. *Independent inquiry into inequalities in health.* Acheson Report. London: The Stationery Office, 1998.

5 *Community Health Council regulations* 1996. London: DoH, S.I. 1996 No. 640.

6 Institute of Health Service Management, The NHS Confederation and NHS Executive. *In the public interest: developing a strategy for public participation in the NHS.* London: IHSM, 1998.

7 Association of Community Health Councils for England and Wales. *CHCs making a difference.* London: ACHCEW, 1997.

8 Hogg C. *The public and the NHS.* London: ACHCEW, 1986.

9 Association of Community Health Councils for England and Wales. *CHCs, health authorities and social service departments: accountability and joint working.* London: ACHCEW, 1996.

10 Association of Community Health Councils for England and Wales. *CHCs making our nation healthier.* London: ACHCEW, 1998.

11 NHS Executive. *Health improvement programmes; planning for better health and better healthcare—supporting guidance.* HSC 1998/167. Leeds: NHSE, 1998

12 Barker J, Bullen M, de Ville J. *Reference manual for public involvement.* London: Bromley Health Authority, West Kent Health Authority, Lambeth, Southwark and Lewisham Health Authority, 1997.

▶9

Setting and monitoring clinical standards

Dr Timothy Riley

Head of Clinical Outcomes and Effectiveness, Public Health Development Unit, NHS, Leeds, UK

On 1st July 1998, Frank Dobson, Secretary of State for Health, launched the consultation document *A First Class Service*[(1)], which signalled a focus on quality in the NHS. Quality had already been identified as a key Government commitment in the December 1997 white paper, *The New NHS*[(2)], by stating that there should be 'a shift of focus onto quality of care'.

The consultation document marks the start of a 10-year programme for improving healthcare quality. Fundamental to this approach is the need to define clear standards of service, dependable local delivery and the monitoring of standards. At each stage, patients and users of the service will be involved.

New mechanisms to define, set and monitor clinical standards

Two new mechanisms have been proposed to enable clinical and service standards to be defined and set:

- National Institute for Clinical Excellence (NICE)
- national service frameworks (NSFs).

To monitor these standards, two further mechanisms will be critical:

- performance assessment framework
- Commission for Health Improvement (CHI).

NICE is a new, special health authority of the NHS and will act as a nationwide appraisal body for new and existing treatments and disseminate consistent advice on what does and does not work. The NSFs will set out the common standards for the treatment of particular conditions.

NICE will play a key role in the development of best clinical advice by undertaking appraisal and by developing guidance—in each case having carefully considered the implications for clinical practice of the evidence on clinical and cost-effectiveness. NICE will also disseminate the guidance and develop and disseminate supporting audit methodologies. Appraisal is a newly recognized function as, until now, there has been no coherent approach to the appraisal of research evidence.

Why is a national approach needed?

In the absence of a systematic approach to appraisal of research evidence, guidance has been developed and issued by numerous bodies at national, regional and local levels. Each of these has adopted different approaches to appraising the evidence and to the standards adopted in their guidance. This has been confusing to clinicians, managers and patients alike. NICE will provide a single national focus of appraisal and guidance and consistency to standard setting. No longer will there be reason for duplication of activity as NICE will progressively replace the appraisal function currently being carried out by the regional development and evaluation committees and other regional and local groups. The programme for NICE will be agreed with the Department of Health and will be driven by information emerging from horizon scanning and by the development of the NSFs and other major NHS priorities (including *Our Healthier Nation*[3]).

The guidance from NICE will include guidelines for the management of certain diseases or conditions and the appropriate use of particular interventions. NICE guidance will cover all aspects of the management of a condition—from self-care through to primary and secondary care and more specialist services. Guidance, in particular on drugs and/or devices, will be developed with the involvement of the various relevant industries which will need to enhance their capacity to produce the necessary evidence of clinical and cost-effectiveness. When a product comes to market without clinical and cost-effectiveness evidence, then NICE may recommend that the NHS should initially channel use of that product through protocol-driven and controlled research. In this way, patients can be assured of the benefit of treatments used widely throughout the NHS.

Implementation of guidelines

A range of tools exists to encourage the implementation of clinical guidance. These include:

- clinical audit programmes
- local prescribing policies
- formularies and guidelines
- lifelong learning.

With NICE as a focus for these initiatives, health authorities will be expected to designate *lead clinicians* to have responsibility for leading the implementation process. Effective dissemination will be crucial to ensure that not only those in the NHS get the best tools and information to improve quality, but that users and patients also get the information they need.

Clinical audit is the key

Clinical audit is a key component of effective implementation. While NICE will not be directly involved in monitoring itself, it will develop the audit tools for use locally through clinical governance. NICE will also, through its work on clinical standards, inform the development of indicators to be implemented through the new national performance assessment framework[4].

Alongside the performance assessment framework with its emphasis on outcomes and standards, there will be complementary approaches to monitoring, including professional self-regulation (employing audit tools) and the independent scrutiny of implementation provided by the CHI. The CHI will conduct systematic service reviews in which it will follow through the implementation of NSFs and NICE guidelines. Clinical governance variations from expected good practice, as recommended by NICE, will increasingly be challenged locally so that the overall impact will be of best practice advice implemented consistently across the NHS.

Conclusions

With their new, focused role on strategy, quality and development, health authorities will take the lead in identifying, implementing and monitoring clinical standards to achieve high-quality service delivery for health and healthcare. The national initiatives for setting and monitoring the standards (NICE, CHI, performance assessment framework) are designed to support health authorities and the rest of the NHS in delivering standards to improve their population's health.

Key messages

- *The New NHS* has emphasized the shift of focus onto quality of care
- Health authorities have a duty to identify, implement and monitor the standards of care planned and delivered to their populations
- The single national focus through NICE will avoid duplication and confusion and ensure acceptability by clinicians and equity in service delivery
- A national approach will help to reduce the variations in clinical standards across the NHS
- A range of tools exists to encourage the implementation of the clinical standards and guidance.

References

1 Department of Health. *A first class service: quality in the new NHS.* London: Department of Health, 1998.

2 Secretary of State for Health. *The new NHS: modern and dependable.* London: The Stationery Office, 1997.

3 Secretary of State for Health. *Our healthier nation: a contract for health.* London: The Stationery Office, 1998.

4 NHS Executive. *A national framework for assessing performance.* Leeds: NHSE, 1998.

▶10

Quality: assessment of performance and health outcomes

Dr Azim Lakhani

Director, National Centre for Health Outcomes Development, London School of Hygiene and Tropical Medicine, London, and Institute of Health Sciences, Oxford, UK

This paper highlights issues relating to quality and performance assessment in the context of health improvement programmes (HImPs) and suggests ways in which they may be addressed. If the prime purpose of HImPs is to use available resources to achieve the greatest improvement in health, then the extent to which this has been achieved is a question for performance assessment.

The Government consultation document *A First Class Service*[(1)] sets out three aspects of a strategy to drive the improvement of performance in the NHS by:

- setting clear standards
- delivering standards by promoting effective delivery of high-quality services locally
- monitoring standards by ensuring that there are strong monitoring mechanisms in place externally.

Performance assessment is central to all of these activities. *A First Class Service*[(1)] highlighted the need for a performance framework which would support the drive for higher quality standards. *The NHS Performance Assessment Framework*[(2)], published following a consultation exercise, describes six areas of performance:

- *Health improvement:* to reflect the umbrella aims of improving the general health of the population and of reducing health inequalities, which are influenced by many factors reaching well beyond the NHS
- *Fair access:* to recognize that the NHS contribution must begin with offering fair access to its services in relation to people's needs, irrespective of geography, socioeconomic group, ethnicity, age or gender
- *Effective delivery of appropriate healthcare:* to recognize that the fair access must be to care that is effective, appropriate, timely and complies with agreed standards
- *Efficiency:* to ensure that the effective care is delivered with a minimum of waste and that the NHS uses its resources to achieve value for money
- *Patient and carer experience:* to assess the way in which patients and their carers experience and view the quality of the care they receive, to ensure that the NHS is sensitive to individual needs
- *Health outcomes of NHS care:* to assess the direct contribution of NHS care to improvements in overall health and complete the circle back to the umbrella goal of health improvement.

Each of the six areas may be divided further into more specific performance aspects. For example, health outcomes of NHS care are described in terms of success in using resources to:

- promote health
- reduce levels of risk factors
- reduce levels of diseases and impairment
- reduce complications of treatment
- improve quality of life for patients and carers
- reduce premature death.

Monitoring achievement in relation to standards set for each of the six areas may be achieved either through the production of comparative data at national level or measurement at local level. This paper will show how this has been attempted in the NHS in England over a number of years in the context of two of the performance assessment areas—health improvement and health outcomes of NHS care.

Challenges

Any serious attempt at addressing the kinds of questions listed within the health improvement and outcomes sections of the performance framework pose a number of challenges relating to:

- concepts
- technical issues
- uses and usefulness of data.

Concepts

All the concepts described below have implications for the monitoring of success.

- *Definitions*: The first challenge relates to varying definitions for and levels of understanding of the term 'outcome'. Some regard 'health outcome' as a state of health or wellbeing at a point in time. Others regard it as a change in state, although, for example, there may not be much change in the level of physical disability from one point in time to another. This may still be considered a positive outcome as the alternative might have been a deterioration in the level of disability. Yet others consider outcome as a result (an attributable effect). This requires measurement not just of the health state or change but also its attribution to intervention. Yet others define outcome as a benefit, given that the objectives of the NHS are to offer benefit. Here, success would be measured in terms of the benefit actually achieved. It is important to have common understanding and agreement of definitions as this will influence the way in which success is judged.
- *Types of outcome*: There are different kinds of outcomes, ie health outcomes, economic outcomes, etc. The type of outcome being measured needs to be specified. If it is to be measured in terms of 'health', then this raises a new set of issues. For example, disease and ill health may be measured in terms of:
  - a biological state, eg biochemical changes in the blood
  - physical impairment, eg blindness
  - clinical signs and symptoms, eg swelling or tenderness
  - function, eg mobility
  - feeling of wellbeing
  - impact on quality of life.

- *Outcomes as results*: If outcome is described as a result, then it may be important to state what it is a result of. A state of health may be a result of healthcare intervention but may also result from lack of timely intervention. Examples include treatment of high blood pressure and the avoidance of stroke. Figure 10.1 shows variation between populations of NHS Executive Regional Offices in overall levels of high blood pressure as well as treated and controlled high blood pressure[(3)]. In some cases a particular health state may be the collective result of the natural history of a health problem and the results of healthcare, social care and wider efforts of society. Attribution may thus be very complicated. In other cases there may be little that the health services can do and a particular health endpoint may be inevitable. Thus, when an outcome is meant to reflect a result, it is very important to understand the extent to which that particular state of health is amenable to change. Health outcomes as results should be measured in the context of specific health outcome objectives, based on an understanding from scientific evaluation of interventions of the extent to which such change may be possible.
- *Perspectives*: In choosing which outcome to measure there may be a number of perspectives which may vary between clinicians, patients, carers, public health specialists, commissioners of healthcare, providers of healthcare, service managers, policy-makers, the public, researchers and others. Figure 10.2 shows variation between clinician and patient perspectives based on data from an audit of outcomes of mental health and social care[(4)].

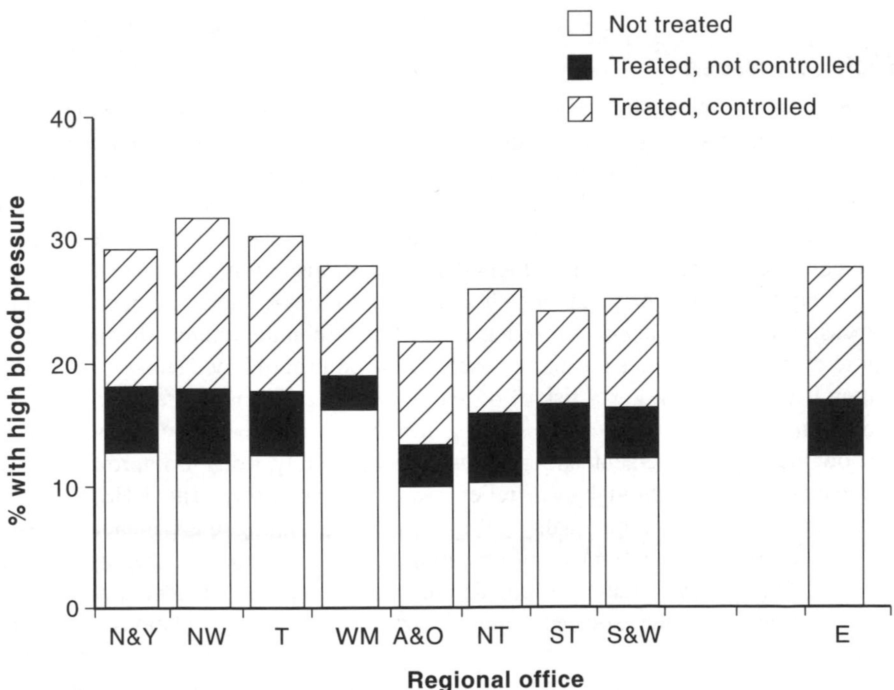

Fig. 10.1 Regional variation in control of high blood pressure in people aged 45–65 years in 1996 ($n = 3989$).

High blood pressure is defined as systolic >160 mmHg and diastolic >95 mmHg. Source: Health Survey for England, National Centre for Health Outcomes Development, 1996. Reproduced with permission.

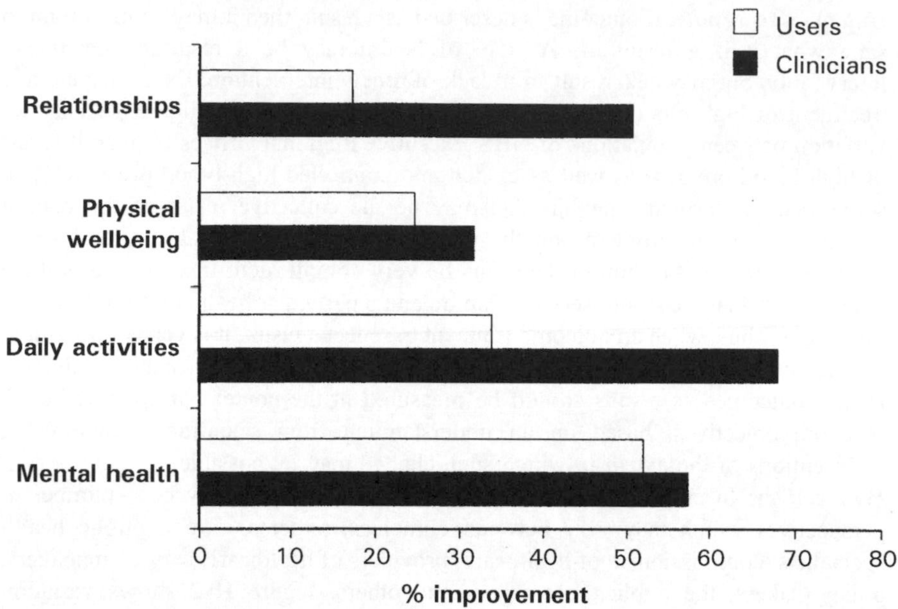

Fig. 10.2 Comparison of user and clinician views on restoring function and improving quality of life in mental health patients.
Source: CORE outcomes study[(4)].

Technical issues

- *Timing short-, medium- and long-term outcomes*: In some cases an outcome may manifest itself soon after a treatment, eg reduced discomfort after treatment for a stomach ulcer. In others it may take many years, eg kidney failure as a complication of untreated diabetes. In the latter case, it may become necessary to use proxy measures for outcome and measures of intermediate states, eg if there is good scientific evidence that control of blood sugar with insulin in patients with diabetes is likely to prevent complications, then the level of appropriate treatment could be measured and act as a proxy in anticipation of benefit in the future. Alternatively, an intermediate change in state may be used, eg the control of blood sugar level, which may itself indicate a lower risk of developing complications in the future.
- *Substitute for improvement in quality of life*: There is research-based evidence to show that hip replacement surgery, if used appropriately, leads to improvements in the quality of life through pain relief and greater mobility. The NHS does not collect data routinely on quality of life outcomes among the patients it treats. However, data on the numbers of operations carried out may be used as a proxy. Figure 10.3 shows variation in population rates of hip replacement as well as an association with the socioeconomic characteristics of populations—deprived populations appear to be getting less of this potentially beneficial treatment[(5)]. This interpretation requires some caution as there are no data on incidence of disease, criteria for selection of patients for surgery, thresholds for treatment, appropriateness of the operation for individual patients, local waiting list initiatives, etc and these may vary between populations.

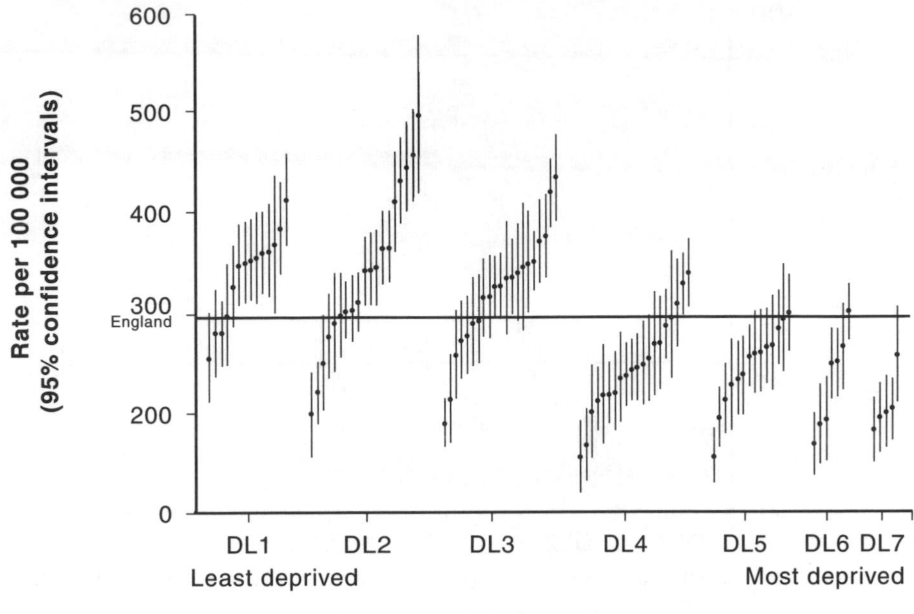

Fig. 10.3 Variation in directly age-standardized rate of primary hip replacement in people aged over 65 years in 1995/96 according to health authority grouped by level of deprivation.
Based on work by Raleigh V and Kiri V using data from the Public Health Common Data Set 1997: PHO-B7.2, PHCDS 1997. Reproduced with permission.

- *Period of measurement*: Outcome measurements may be presented as values at one point in time, across a period of time such as a year, a series of cross-sectional values showing trends over years or as longitudinal measures examining what happens to an individual patient or a group of patients over time. Figure 10.4 shows age- and sex-standardized death rates due to coronary heart disease among people under 65 years of age, resident in 100 health authorities in England, with data pooled for three years[(5)]. The health authorities have been grouped on the basis of a classification of areas developed by the Office for National Statistics enabling the comparison of death rates between populations with similar social and demographic characteristics.
- *Attribution*: This may be very complicated. In many cases a particular state of health is a cumulative endpoint of a whole range of services and interventions. For cxample, a stroke or death following it could be the result of political decisions, environmental issues, patient behaviour, preventive health interventions, primary healthcare, diagnostic services, treatment, emergency care, etc. The context and natural progression of a particular disease may need to be taken into account.
- *Completeness and quality of routine data*: In interpreting outcomes data based on routine statistics, the completeness and quality of the data need to be taken into account. For example, if operations or diagnoses are not coded well in hospital records, then indicators which rely on such codes may show fewer events and would be incomplete.

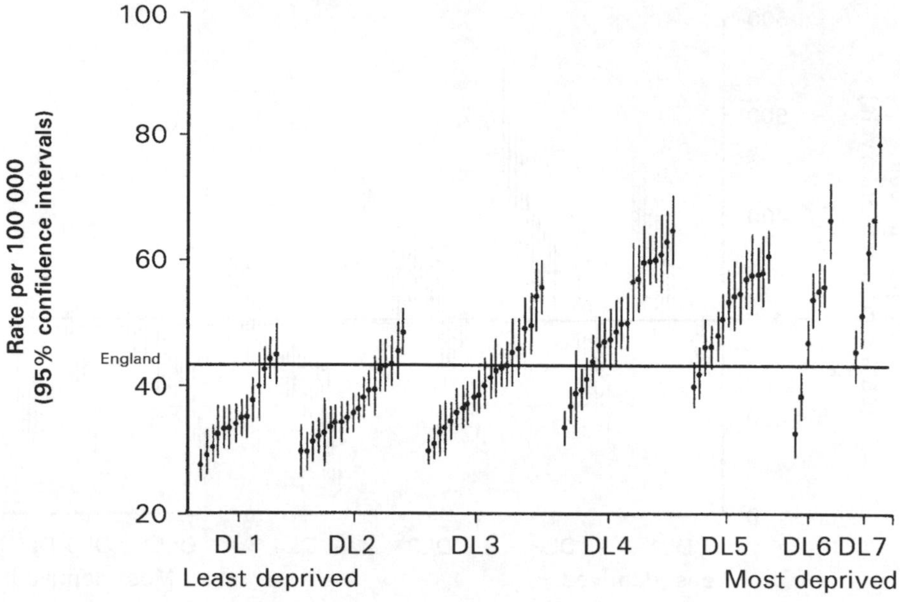

Fig. 10.4 Variation in directly age-standardized mortality rate from coronary heart disease in people aged under 65 years in 1994–96 according to health authority grouped by level of deprivation.

Based on work by Raleigh V and Kiri V using data from the Public Health Common Data Set 1997: HON-A1, PHCDS 1997. Reproduced with permission.

- *Explaining variation in comparative data*: In looking at variation between populations it is important to ensure that the numerators and denominators used to analyse the indicator match as far as is possible. For example, differences between populations in deaths from certain diseases may reflect the level of such diseases in the populations and not necessarily the outcomes of treatment. In addition, some of the variation may be due to chance events, which may vary between populations and from year to year.

Uses of data

- *Different approaches*: While performance should ideally be monitored against stated objectives, targets or standards, these may not exist. An alternative is to produce comparative data. Variation in comparative data may suggest that performance is suboptimal, even in the absence of standards, and could lead to further investigation and uncover problems with service delivery.
- *Central versus local analyses*: Central development of indicators ensures that there is standardization of definitions, numerators and denominators, hence comparability. However, this may reduce choice and flexibility and ownership by those who might end up using the indicators locally. Central production is also dependent on central collation and availability of the data and thus on the speed of the slowest contributor. For example, cancer registration data in England are currently many

years out of date. This also has implications for the timeliness of the publication of indicators and their potential usefulness.

- *Level of aggregation*: There are issues concerning the unit of aggregation within indicators and the numbers making up the indicator values. Meaningful variation may only be detected when numbers are large and hence require analyses at a high level of aggregation, eg whole hospitals or health authorities with large populations. These may, however, mask variations within such organizations and may be too crude for meaningful comparison. Such aggregations may also be too broad for meaningful application at local level although they may show trends which are important and useful at national level. Smaller levels of aggregation, on the other hand, may lead to numbers which are too small for meaningful comparison, with the added risk of identifying individual clinicians and patients.
- *Follow-up work*: Publication of the indicators on their own may have little impact. The role of such indicators in performance management needs to be considered, including the incentives for their use, sanctions available and levers for change.

Options for addressing challenges

Compendium of Clinical and Health Indicators for the NHS in England

The National Centre for Health Outcomes Development, recently set up by the Department of Health in England, has brought together a number of historical nationally produced data sets—the traditional public health common data set, population health outcome indicators, 'Health of the Nation/Our Healthier Nation' indicators, clinical indicators, cancer survival indicators and others—into a single, structured Compendium of Clinical and Health Indicators. This has involved the identification and grouping of indicators by clinical area, eg asthma, stroke, pregnancy and childbirth, as well as removal of overlap, duplication and inconsistency between indicators in the historical data sets. There are currently some 175 indicators and their variants in the Compendium, covering some 40 clinical areas. The Compendium is currently being prepared for publication and will be one source of comparative indicators for the monitoring of health outcomes based on routinely collected data.

Specification of new indicators

In previous work on the development of indicators at national level, the key criterion in the selection of indicators has been the requirement that they be based on routinely collected data. This practical constraint meant that indicators were opportunistic rather than ideal. In an attempt to overcome this, 10 working groups were established to look at specific clinical areas, eg stroke and asthma, to develop new, better indicators and acknowledge that some of these may need new data collection. All relevant clinical professions were represented in each working group, in addition to public health, policy makers, patient representatives, managers, researchers and others as appropriate. The reports of the working groups are being prepared for publication in 1999. The indicators cover a variety of perspectives, eg clinical, patient and carer, and a variety of settings including primary care, hospital, community and health authority.

Overviews

Given the issues described above, it is important that single indicators are not examined in isolation. Figure 10.5 shows how a variety of healthcare activities, resource use and health outcomes may be brought together to provide a broader view of achievements in relation to the management of high blood pressure and stroke. Examination of data just on hospital treatment of stroke or population death rates would provide an incomplete picture. In addition, an overview such as this may raise fundamental questions about value for money in the context of HImPs. The bulk of direct expenditure is weighted towards treatment and long-term care for stroke, a potentially avoidable condition. Figure 10.1 shows that outcomes of preventive services are less than optimal.

Local follow-up work

Following a review of ways in which health authorities in England used population health outcome assessments and indicators, the Wessex Institute for Health Research and Development was commissioned to compile a series of case studies on local work undertaken to follow-up national indicator data and initiatives. A series of 26 studies has been published, giving pragmatic accounts of reasons for undertaking the studies, methods used, results and local action based on the findings[(6)]. Many of

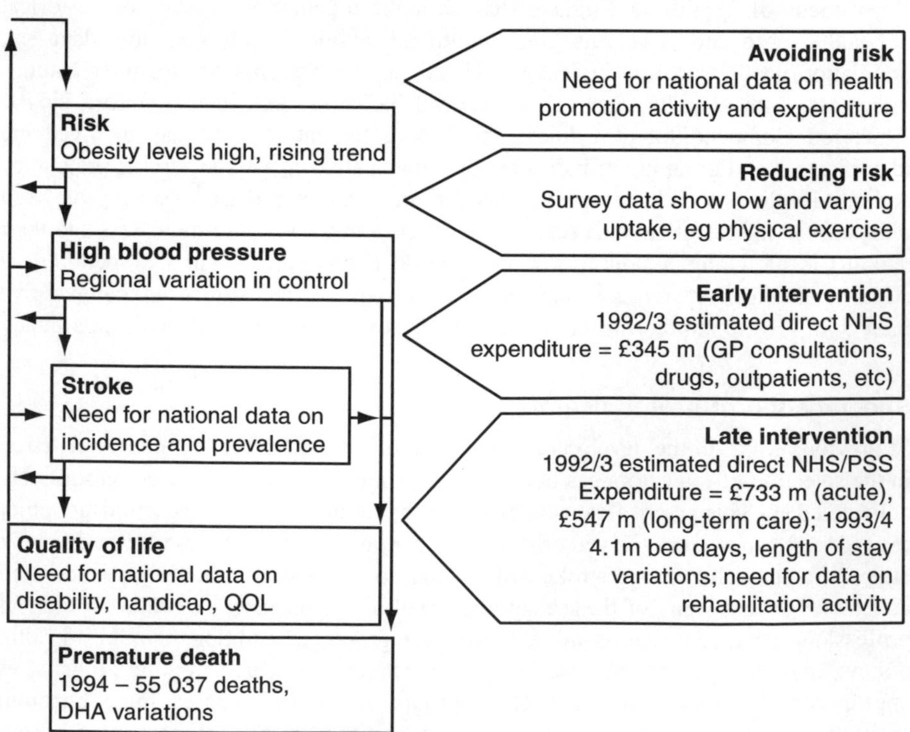

Fig. 10.5 Stroke activity, resource use and outcomes in England.
Source: National Centre for Health Outcomes Development based on various Department of Health publications.

ıalities in access to, and shortcomings in the quality of,

lescribed are not precise measures of outcome but are
ot have been achieved in relation to stated objectives.
ıes for further investigation. Despite their limitations,
y towards helping the NHS and others to judge the
ı successful in its attempts to use its resources to
vement in health. Much more can be done locally
e data and judge performance and outcomes in

to assess the extent to which current
d their objectives (ie outcomes)
service and clinical standards (setting,

all activities
ıeasure of performance but an indicator

based on routine data supplemented
hievements in health improvement.

are those of the author and not necessarily those of the

new NHS. London: DoH, 1998.
vork. Leeds: NHS Executive, 1999.
England 1996. London: The Stationery

. London: BPS Centre for Outcomes,

1997. Surrey: National Institute

case studies on how English
mpton: Wessex Institute fo

►11

Clinical quality: a US perspective

Dr Vivien Chen
Associate Director of Quality Assurance, Department of Health and Human Resources, Washington, USA

The US has gained much knowledge of health service delivery by studying the experiences of the UK. For years, the UK has led the way in providing a model for serving the healthcare needs of its citizens through managed care. In doing so, it has enabled others to learn from its experiences and set their own framework for healthcare provision. Both the UK and the US systems have evolved and found ways to handle national clinical quality issues. The US has adapted aspects of the UK system and created other programmes to meet its public health needs; there are a number of efforts underway to contain costs and mechanisms applied to ensure quality healthcare. Recent efforts in both countries to create clinical quality improvement measures reflect similar trends.

Clinical quality improvement

As in the UK, creating a system of quality healthcare that meets the needs of all people in the US is complex. The changes over the past 10 years in the US health service delivery system have been triggered by the projected oversupply of specialists (eg cardiologists, neurologists, etc) and escalating healthcare costs. The desire to accommodate these changes has led to the evolution and integration of managed care systems, thus creating tension between practitioners and increased pressure from consumers. The primary concern of both groups is whether or not quality of care will be compromised by cost-containment. This has prompted researchers and practitioners to develop national models and studies to evaluate such changes. These efforts are intended to improve health status and ensure quality care while reducing healthcare costs. There are many approaches and special considerations to be made in the development of appropriate models.

As in the UK, there are numerous federal initiatives underway in the US that are beyond the scope of this paper. The most familiar are those designed to address system-wide aspects beginning with primary care education and faculty development to direct service delivery models. There are as many initiatives in the private sector, which is perhaps taking the lead in the development of clinical quality improvement to meet its specific needs. In terms of determining and monitoring actual health improvement, two federal efforts come to mind.

Healthy People 2010

Healthy People 2000[(1)] and the national development of clinical protocol/guidelines, while noteworthy activities, are nationally constructed based on data that meet the needs of majority populations and, for the most part, are not determined with sample sizes reflective of the specific needs of special populations. Fortunately, efforts to develop objectives for 'People 2010'[(2)] are underway and these do take into account some of the special populations and their needs.

The specific needs of special populations and their significance in appropriate modelling must be remembered. As an advocate for equal access, I have always been critical of 'planning oversight' or what I consider poor planning. When attempting to create national health plans, the questions that should always be asked are What are we attempting to achieve? and Who are we trying to help? Historically, most strategies to improve health status have focused on the 80:20 rule rather than population-based or targeted protocols and guidelines. Clearly, there are political and technical reasons for this. While it is important to take care of 80%, ie most, of the population, the remaining 20%, the most disenfranchised, tend to be the most underserved and this is reflected in higher morbidity rates (eg higher cancer rates among certain ethnic and subethnic groups).

Legislation to improve health

Among the many initiatives in the US, three pieces of legislation have been passed as a means of improving healthcare and protecting the public. They attempt to address the monitoring of performance (through peer review), based on adverse actions taken against healthcare practitioners, providers and suppliers. In effect, these reported actions may be considered 'quality data on outlier performance'. The first and second pieces of legislation are the amended *Healthcare Quality Improvement Act of 1986* (42USC 11101–11152) and *Medicare/caid Patient and Programme Protection Acts of 1987* (42 USC 13961–2, 104 Stat 1388–208–209), which are both means of improving peer-review efforts, examining medical malpractice costs, and enabling tracking of problem practitioners from state to state. The 1996 passage of the *Health Insurance Portability and Accountability Act* (42USC 1320a–7e, 110 Stat 2009–2011) was an effort to reduce escalating healthcare costs caused by fraud and abuse. The collection of such data is intended to be used as a flagging system for 'credentialing' and peer review.

Title IV of Public Law 99-660 (Healthcare Quality Improvement Act of 1986)

The passage of this Act resulted from the growing concern over increased medical malpractice litigation and the weaknesses in medical peer review. It led to the establishment of the National Practitioners Data Bank (NPDB) which collects information on adverse actions based on quality concerns taken against physicians and dentists and medical malpractice payments made for, or on behalf of, all healthcare practitioners. It also contains adverse professional society membership actions against physicians and dentists.

The legislation requires information to be reported by medical malpractice payers, Boards of Medical/Dental Examiners, professional societies with formal peer review and hospitals and healthcare entities. Other healthcare entities, the practitioners (self-query only) and researchers (reports devoid of all identifiers) may request information;

the case studies show inequalities in access to, and shortcomings in the quality of, service delivery.

Conclusions

The approaches and indicators described are not precise measures of outcome but are indicative of what may or may not have been achieved in relation to stated objectives. They also raise questions and issues for further investigation. Despite their limitations, official statistics may go some way towards helping the NHS and others to judge the extent to which the NHS has been successful in its attempts to use its resources to achieve the greatest possible improvement in health. Much more can be done locally to supplement national comparative data and judge performance and outcomes in HImPs.

Key messages

- The starting point for HImP is to assess the extent to which current programmes/services have achieved their objectives (ie outcomes)
- Improving performance is about service and clinical standards (setting, delivering and monitoring standards)
- Performance assessment is central to all activities
- Outcome indicators are not a precise measure of performance but an indicator for further questions and investigations
- Despite limitations, outcome measures based on routine data supplemented with local data will help in assessing achievements in health improvement.

Acknowledgement

This work was funded by the Department of Health. All views expressed are those of the author and not necessarily those of the Department of Health.

References

1 Department of Health. *A first class service—quality in the new NHS.* London: DoH, 1998.
2 NHS Executive. *The NHS performance assessment framework.* Leeds: NHS Executive, 1999.
3 Prescott-Clarke P, Primatesta P, eds. *Health survey for England 1996.* London: The Stationery Office, 1998.
4 Clifford P. *Outcomes audit of the care programme approach.* London: BPS Centre for Outcomes, Research and Effectiveness, 1999.
5 Department of Health. *Public health common data set 1997.* Surrey: National Institute of Epidemiology, 1997.
6 McColl A, Roderick P, Gabbay J. *Improving health outcomes—case studies on how English health authorities use population health outcome assessments.* Southampton: Wessex Institute for Health Research and Development, 1997.

Boards of Medical/Dental Examiners and other healthcare practitioner state licensing boards may request information for the purpose of licensing and 'credentialing' only. Information is confidential and may only be used for the purpose for which it is disclosed. Other provisions of the legislation are that:

- the hospitals are obliged to question practitioners when granting privileges, and every two years thereafter; and granting immunity for damages arising from civil suits
- the information is not shared but used for the sole purposes for which it is intended.

Section 1921 of the Social Security Act of 1987

In 1987, Section 1921 of the Social Security Act, as amended by Section 5(b) of the Medicare and Medicaid Patient and Programme Protection Act of 1987, Public Law 100–93 and the Omnibus Budget Reconciliation Act of 1990, Public Law 101-508, was passed. This Act broadened efforts to collect information on adverse actions to actions taken against *all* licensed practitioners and entities. The legislation also enabled the collection of peer-review organizations' (PROs) actions and private accreditation actions. More specifically, it enabled the NPDB to include adverse licensure actions and other negative actions or findings against healthcare practitioners and entities, licensed or otherwise authorized by a state to provide healthcare services. This information will be disclosed to:

- agencies administering federal healthcare programmes
- state Medicaid fraud control units
- utilization and quality-control peer-review groups
- certain law enforcement officials.

Information is confidential and may be used only for the purpose for which it is disclosed.

Public Law 104-191 (Health Insurance Portability and Accountability Act of 1996)

In 1996, Public Law 104-191, The Health Insurance Portability and Accountability Act was passed in an effort to reduce escalating healthcare costs in fraud and abuse. This new data collection system mandated in this legislation will contain all final adverse action taken against all licensed practitioners, providers and suppliers. Adverse action data include healthcare-related criminal convictions and civil judgements, federal and state licensing and certification actions, exclusions from federal and state healthcare programmes and certain other final adjudicated adverse actions or decisions against healthcare practitioners, providers and suppliers, including business organizations and facilities. Federal and state agencies and health plans are required to report. They may request this information for the purpose of 'credentialing' licensing, claim/fraud investigation and other related activities. Information is confidential and may be used only for the purpose for which it is disclosed.

Can legislation improve clinical quality?

The key question is, how can these efforts create clinical quality improvement models? I believe that, since the passage of the above legislation, most of the data collected in these data systems reflect the outlier data of clinical outcomes[3]. Without discussing the complexities of medical malpractice and the politics involved in taking a final adverse action against a practitioner (and thus being reported), the data are representative of actions taken nationally when a disciplinary action is taken or medical malpractice payment is made. It can also be said that the data represented are reliable and valid.

Such data reflect valuable indicators where a failure may have occurred and are coded according to the type of action taken, cost, description of the act or omission and reason (eg missed or improper diagnosis). The information identifies the type of practitioner and events that led to the 'failure'. When using these data, it must be recognized that the likelihood of any of these events occurring is generally limited and, therefore, the database is relatively small when looking for a pattern of a specific event occurring in an institution. However, the utility of the data when aggregated can provide insight into areas in which unintended events are occurring and in which resources are being expended.

If these data are to be used for internal clinical quality improvement efforts, a number of systems improvements can be implemented (eg replacing the narrative fields with codified data elements where mandatory data elements are requested or improving the data by coding the severity of the event, specialty, etc).

Professional organizations responsible for the monitoring or training of health professionals can use the data to examine the outlier patterns in their professional category to determine continuing education needs.

The challenges

The UK continues to examine ways of establishing quality improvement models but to be successful a commitment is required to provide the necessary resources to support the development of and data collection for a data-tracking system. The education of policy makers and clinicians is also required if they are to understand the importance of data in programme planning, reducing costs and overcoming the fear of working with data as a management tool.

The greatest challenges are in:

- creating the interest and skills to provide the information
- application across disciplines (alternative medicine), populations and diseases
- the implementation and creation of appropriate prevention/clinical practice improvement models through the population-based data.

It is also important to emphasize a few key, and by no means easy, tasks:

- Know what you need and who are you really trying to reach. If data are to be collected, determine what you need and overcome the general fear in data collection
- Data must be population-based. It should contain specialty and severity codes and be ethnic/subethnic relevant for health planning and protocol/guideline development.

- Data must account for demographic shifts
- Data, especially when the sample size is small, are more meaningful and useful when developing health plans and protocols for local areas
- When developing quality improvement models or protocol/guidelines, national data can be used but local data must be applied for greater specificity
- Commitment, patience and time (resources): change in attitude and behaviour must be achieved at all (management and practitioner) levels
- Re-emphasis of patient care provided through medical ethics training and the Hippocratic oath—Who are you treating and what is the goal?
- The model must be simple, practical and inclusive to meet the needs of the entire community. It will require community involvement.

Conclusions

To change the way data are used in improving healthcare is by no means an easy undertaking, nor is it always easy to assess the complete picture without total commitment. I have provided examples of ways in which the US has legislated quality assurance efforts that are ultimately to assist in protecting the public and improving peer-review activities. The data collected, primarily adverse actions, represent outlier healthcare indicators. These health outliers are the result of unintended outcomes and cost the healthcare system time and money to resolve. Such indicators should be considered part of the entire 'gestalt' of healthcare and be included in the development of clinical improvement efforts.

Many argue that adverse actions are not great predictors or indicators of healthcare and are an administrative burden to collect. However, they do reflect the severity, diagnosis and outcome of a given event that leads to an adverse action against the provider. Only by changing thinking about the type of data needed and examining the entire system in greater detail can there be success in improving the entire healthcare system and in reducing its costs. Swimming against the mainstream is not always easy but possible when swimming together to achieve quality improvement.

Key messages

- US efforts are intended to improve health status and ensure quality care while reducing healthcare costs
- A legislative framework was used as a means of improving healthcare and protecting the public from medical malpractice
- Specific laws were designed to collect data on adverse actions (eg disciplinary actions and malpractice payments), peer reviews, fraud and abuse
- Data collected on disciplinary action or malpractice can be valuable indicators of where a failure has occurred
- While these data represent outlier patterns, they nevertheless provide a valuable tool for monitoring and training to improve quality of care.

References

1 *Healthy people 2000, national health promotion, disease prevention objectives*. Washington: US Department of Health and Human Services, Public Health Service, Publication no PHS91-50212, Feb 1991.

2 *Healthy people 2010*. Draft for public comment, proposed objectives. http://web.health.gov/healthy people.

3 Horn SD. *Clinical practice improvement methodology: implementation, evaluation, medical outcomes and practice guidelines*. Library II, vol II. New York: Faulkner & Gray, 1997.

▶ 12

Medical schools, universities and health improvement programmes: getting the balance right

Professor Robert Boyd
Principal, St George's Hospital Medical School, London, UK

> 'In a complicated state of society in large towns, death, as everyone of great experience knows, is far less often produced by any one organic disease than by some illness after many other diseases producing just the sum of exhaustion necessary for death.'
>
> 'It is well known that the same names may be seen constantly recurring on workhouse books for generations... death and disease are like the workhouse: they take from the same family, the same house or, in other words, the same conditions. Why will we not observe what they are?'
>
> 'The causes of the enormous child mortality are perfectly well known... the remedies are just as well known; and among them is certainly not the establishment of a child's hospital.'
>
> (Florence Nightingale, *Notes on Nursing*, 1859)

The agenda for health improvement of the citizens of a locality should have three interrelated elements:

- Reduction of their poverty, improvement of morale and change in lifestyle
- Enrichment (from clean water to social cohesion) of the economic, social, physical and cultural environment in which they live and its technical and wider capacity to reduce their burden of disease and disability
- Increasing the ability of its health professionals (widely interpreted to include medicine, nursing, social work, professions allied to medicine [PAMs] and others) to work in partnership with the citizens and each other; their professional skill and skill mix and their numbers, deployment and coherence as a local team.

To be effective, each of these elements must be based on an underpinning and evolving archive of knowledge and scholarship based on research. This chapter will consider predominately education and its interaction with the third of these three elements but universities and their NHS clinical partners can and should contribute directly or indirectly to all three through scholarship and as employers and inner-city beacons, as well as through education. They will make these contributions more effectively if they look resolutely outwards into their local communities, as well as towards their national and international peers, and encourage a positive attitude towards the health improvement programme (HImP) and its staffing, staff development and research needs. Conversely, the ability to mount a successful HImP at the local level depends critically on the locality's ability to recruit and retain able staff. Recruitment and retention, especially in challenging environments, is more likely to be achieved if the local university is strong. Local communities and their health leadership should therefore work to ensure that this is the case. To be so, the university's various roles must be kept in balance.

Four roles of higher education

Universities and their health, social work and medical schools (sadly, often split between different universities) have at least four functions, all of which are challenging.

Education

This includes not just the first qualification, but lifelong learning starting in the immediate postgraduate years and continuing throughout full-time working life and even beyond retirement. Attractiveness to school leavers and mature entrants is critical to recruitment. Recruitment into many health-related professions other than medicine is very competitive in the sense that alternative and exciting opportunities in new or historically male-dominated fields, such as computer science and business studies, are now open to women who still provide 80% of recruits to most branches of healthcare. Teenage girls are now more numerate than boys. Unless these schools continue to attract girls and women and increasingly recruit boys and men, health will have a catastrophic workforce shortfall.

Courses and their clinical elements also need to be educationally strong. They and their regulators need to allow and encourage mature entry, career change, recognition of previous experience and other practices which support recruitment and retention of a wide range of individuals. Education must also respect the diversity of goals students have within the broad church of vocational education from frontline service to laboratory research.

Research and development

R&D is also competitive between institutions. Failure to succeed in the competition at national and international level, especially in medicine, can seriously challenge both institutional financial viability in the long term and, more immediately, the school's ability to recruit and retain the best staff and, perhaps, good quality students.

Clinical service

Provision of direct healthcare and leadership in service innovation by university-employed clinical staff is important, especially in medical schools. Clinical academics provide a major component of the consultant staffing of teaching hospitals. They also work as consultants in public health and as principals in general practice. Although there are stresses in delivering this clinical role[(1)], the clinical academic has been, and remains, a critical cross-link in ensuring that medical schools and professional leadership are able to respond to the needs of the service. Development of a similar approach to the academic structure for other health-related professions is highly desirable.

Contribution to the wider local community

Universities are often important foci of employment and resources of culture and citizen commitment in depressed areas[(2)].

An academic—NHS continuum

In 1997, a former Minister, Lord Glenarthur made the unwise claim that we must not allow 'academic institutions to be the tail that wags the health service dog'[(3)]. To my mind this is a misunderstanding of the joint role of the universities and NHS in providing good quality healthcare and health improvement both *now* and in the long-term *future* (Figure 12.1). The continuum should take the form of a holistic animal—both tail and body! Any healthcare system has to balance current delivery and long-term capacity. In the UK, predominant responsibility for the former lies with the NHS and for the latter with the universities, but neither can function without the other. For success they must work seamlessly together.

Healthcare systems are labour-intensive. Long-term service capacity, quality and improvement therefore depend overwhelmingly on the joint system's success in developing its human resources. These are very long-term issues. A young person choosing his or her sixth form courses today with the intention of becoming a doctor will be retiring under current arrangements in 2049. If, as seems likely, the demographic imperative leads to longer working lives, that individual will be clinically active in the second half of the next century.

Developing the teaching workforce and curricula

Similar long-term issues apply to developing the teaching workforce. To achieve success the joint system needs to recruit and retain students *and* staff of quality who will learn effectively, work hard, share their knowledge and skills with each other and do so in a reflective way which will help them to re-learn and develop over a

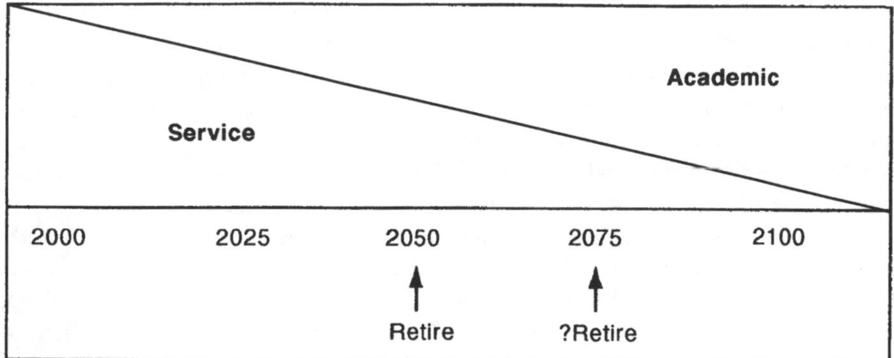

Fig. 12.1 Holistic medicine: the academic and service continuum.
Relations across the line between the two are guided by 10 Key Principles[(4)] and a Joint Declaration[(5)]. Note the short-term dominance of service balanced by the long-term contribution of academia (education and research) as an individual entering in 1998 moves through to retirement mid-century.

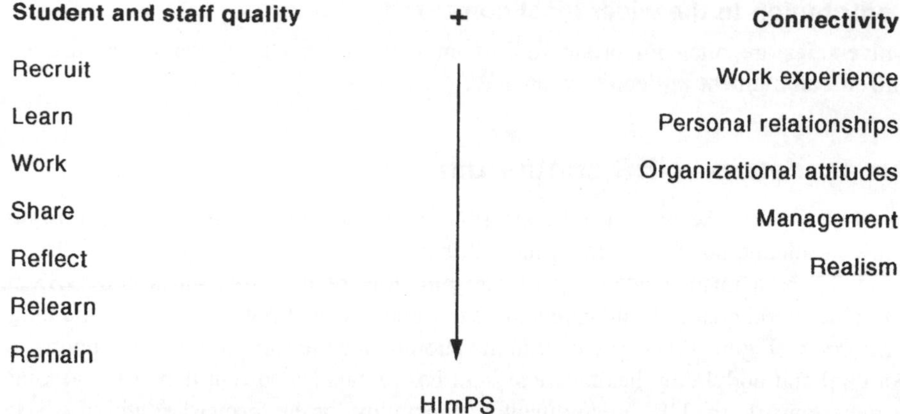

Fig. 12.2 Factors influencing staff and student quality and the ways in which they connect with the 'local health economy' thus contributing to HImPs.

professional lifetime. To contribute to the future health improvement agenda, the student also needs to be imbued with a vocationalism that will inspire him or her to work and enjoy working in the often uninviting communities in most need of help. This is most likely to be achieved through curricula which include clinical placements for students and which provide work experience in needy communities under the guidance of enthusiastic and committed staff. This is clearly a joint NHS—university endeavour with a strong primary care element which needs to be supported by good personal relationships between clinicians and managers in the service and in the school (Figure 12.2). This should also relate to the specific local environment.

Curricula, at least in medicine, have been developed over the last decade with space for such partnerships. Indeed, in *Tomorrow's Doctors*, the General Medical Council recommends a number of reforms to improve fitness for purpose of medical graduates, several of which are relevant to health improvement (Table 12.1)[(6)]. In particular, the diminution of curricular overload with the introduction of special study modules means that students have more opportunity to study some element of social deprivation practically and in depth. More use should probably be made of this. Increased emphasis on communication skills, on understanding public health issues and on the primary care agenda is also helpful. The GMC recommendations provide full opportunity for this and most schools, including my own, have substantially increased general practice and community placements and teaching, communications skills focus and better integration of relevant public health into their courses.

The long-term success of new curricula remains to be demonstrated although early anecdotal reports are positive. We have to be cautious, however, that the scientific content of medicine and the need to learn key clinical skills is not undervalued. Medical graduates from these new courses should be well suited to contribute to HImPs, but medical graduates alone are unlikely to make a substantial impact unless interprofessional teamwork can be taken forward effectively. In the case of other professions there are concerns about clinical skills and a wide perception that more needs to be done[(7)].

Table 12.1 Principal recommendations from Tomorrow's Doctors[6]

1. The **burden of factual information** imposed on students in undergraduate medical curricula should be reduced substantially.
2. **Learning** through curiosity, the exploration of knowledge and the critical evaluation of evidence should be promoted and should ensure a capacity for self-education; the undergraduate course should be seen as the first stage in the continuum of medical education that extends throughout professional life.
3. **Attitudes** of mind and of behaviour that befit a doctor should be inculcated, and should imbue the new graduate with attributes appropriate to his/her future responsibilities to patients, colleagues and society in general.
4. The **essential skills** required by the graduate at the beginning of the pre-registration year must be acquired under supervision, and proficiency in these skills must be assessed rigorously.
5. A **'core curriculum'** encompassing the essential knowledge and skills and the appropriate attitudes that need to be acquired by graduation should be defined.
6. The '*core curriculum*' should be augmented by a series of **'special study modules'** which allow students to study areas of particular interest to them in depth, which provide them with insight into scientific method and the discipline of research, and which engender an approach to medicine that is both questioning and self-critical.
7. The 'core curriculum' should be **system-based**, its component parts being the combined responsibility of basic scientists and clinicians **integrating** their contributions to a common purpose, thus eliminating the rigid pre-clinical–clinical divide and the exclusive departmen- tally based course.
8. There should be emphasis throughout the course on **communication skills** and the other essentials of basic clinical method.
9. The theme of **public health medicine** should figure prominently in the curriculum, encompassing health promotion and illness prevention, assessment and targeting of population needs, and awareness of environmental and social factors in disease.
10. Clinical teaching should adapt to **changing patterns in healthcare** and should provide experience of primary care and of community medical services as well as of hospital-based services.
11. **Learning systems** should be informed by modern educational theory and should draw on the wide range of technological resources available; medical schools should be prepared to share these resources to their mutual advantage.
12. **Assessment systems** should be adapted to the new-style curriculum, should encourage appropriate learning skills and should reduce emphasis on the uncritical acquisition of facts.

Interprofessionalism

Most observers would agree that interprofessional dysfunction in both education and clinical service exists. Old, implicit class and gender systems of professional relationships, with the doctor as male leader and other health professionals as female subordinates, have long gone but have been incompletely replaced by working relationships appropriate to the 21st century: current boundaries between professions seem too high, the role of different professions too fixed and career progression between them too difficult for a rapidly evolving society.

Professional self-identity as a means of maintaining morale, preserving standards and improving technical skills has its place, but the disadvantage of high professional boundaries are all too obvious. There are, of course, excellent examples of clinical teamwork but they stand out by exception rather than the rule. Tribalism all too often leads to complacency and overemphasis of differences. At best, the role of different professionals is confusing to users, especially in deprived communities, and even to other professionals. At worst, the differences can lead to a client no longer being at the centre, which is most sharply illustrated by the debate as to whether a 'social bath' is the duty of the NHS or of local authority staff and by overt rivalries when, for example, members of one profession blame another for disco-ordination and ineffectiveness of service which may be the fault of neither.

These difficulties are accentuated by the different histories, locations and funding of health professions and their recruits. Figure 12.3 indicates the great differences in student recruitment, staff management, funding and career outturn between nursing and medicine; PAMs are different again. Nevertheless, it is heartening to note that school children appear to distinguish less sharply between nursing and medicine as professions than health professionals do[8].

Our limited experience of social interaction between medical students at St George's and the students of other health professions in a faculty of healthcare sciences we share with Kingston University is generally very positive. The provisional

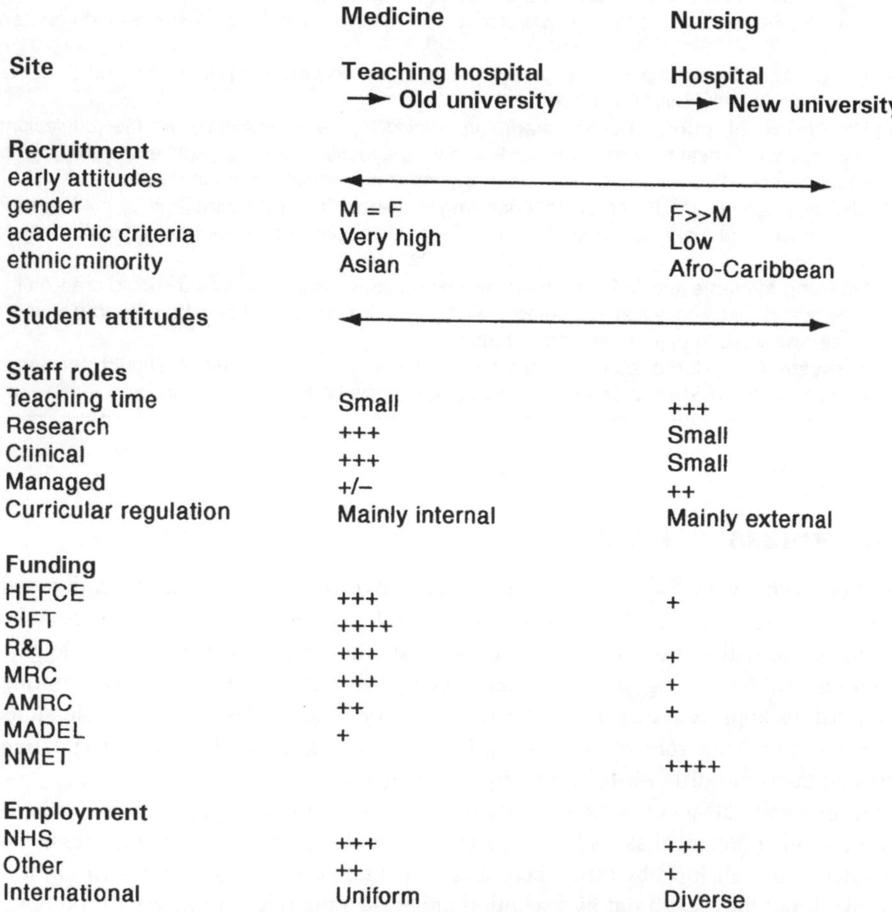

	Medicine	**Nursing**
Site	**Teaching hospital → Old university**	**Hospital → New university**
Recruitment		
early attitudes	←———————————	———————————→
gender	M = F	F>>M
academic criteria	Very high	Low
ethnic minority	Asian	Afro-Caribbean
Student attitudes	←———————————	———————————→
Staff roles		
Teaching time	Small	+++
Research	+++	Small
Clinical	+++	Small
Managed	+/–	++
Curricular regulation	Mainly internal	Mainly external
Funding		
HEFCE	+++	+
SIFT	++++	
R&D	+++	+
MRC	+++	+
AMRC	++	+
MADEL	+	
NMET		++++
Employment		
NHS	+++	+++
Other	++	+
International	Uniform	Diverse

Fig. 12.3 Differences between medicine and nursing in higher education in England.

impressions of a common foundation module shared by all our medical, physiotherapy and radiography students for the first time in 1998 are also encouraging. We anticipate that such developments should give health professionals a better understanding of each other's roles. In the longer term, they may lead to a more cost-effective skill mix in the healthcare team and to better working by the team.

Universities need to replace the interprofessional paternalism of the early 20th century and the separatism of its later decades with a balanced interprofessional partnership, both in education and the approach to research. A capacity for research needs to be developed in all professions without unnecessary and damaging separatism.

Constraints on university contributions to HImPs

There are thus many common interests but also some real short-term conflicts of interest in bringing universities and the NHS together in support of HImPs. These can be minimized if it is accepted that when choosing priorities for investment there is a need to balance the following.

Local versus national or international needs

Local programmes require a range of skills. Making an academic contribution at the international level usually requires deep specialization in a limited area of clinical or public health and its associated science, whether biological or behavioural.

Individual flexibility versus managerialism

Research success for the university depends on the individuals who work there. Forcing talented staff to focus on short-term issues not at the centre of their interest is not the best route to recruiting and retaining the excellent. The possibly tempting alternative of separating research and teaching would run counter to the correct concept of lifelong career development for those working in an industry which, as healthcare does, lies at the vortex of three revolutions—bioscience, information technology and social mores. Far from reducing research and its associated capacity for change, it needs to be extended more vigorously to the non-medical elements of healthcare.

External accountability versus local agenda

All universities in the periodic research assessment exercise (RAE)—next due in 2001—face external peer review of research quality. Schools that do not score highly not only lose money but also prestige. I do not share the belief of some that the most important research is done in those schools with the highest RAE ratings or the general complacency that repeated RAEs have benefited UK academic life[9]. These ratings have certainly increased role conflict between the clinical and research duties of clinical academics and between their local and (inter)national scholarly contributions. Teaching hospitals and other NHS bodies supporting research will be subject to similar national review in the next competitive 'Culyer' funding review in 2000. Those local health economies that score badly may lose substantial funds. An entirely new external review of teaching quality (TQA) is now also in progress. It is too early to say whether or not this will be a beneficial or damaging exercise in the long term.

Whatever their rights and wrongs, RAE, Culyer and TQA success are certainly important if schools *and* their NHS partners are to maintain their prestige and funding and thus their capacity to recruit good individuals into the local health economy; this is an essential first step if schools are to make a full contribution to health improvement although not of course, in itself, sufficient. Clinical governance is a further regulatory pressure that might become counterproductive.

Constraints of different funding mechanisms

The complexity of the major funding streams for health education and research is challenging. The main ones are shown in Table 12.2 and include contributions from Government through its Department for Education and Employment (Higher Education Funding Council), Department of Health (NHS funding) and Office of Science and Technology (Medical Research Council [MRC] and other research councils). Members of the Association of Medical Research Charities (AMRC), such as the Wellcome Trust and British Heart Foundation, jointly spend substantially more than the MRC. The pharmaceutical industry is also a major contributor to research in the NHS and universities. In contrast, the flexibility of funding for nursing and most PAMs is very limited, which makes it difficult to contribute the time of those involved in nurse and PAM education to research or clinical activity—which would, of course, be highly desirable.

The appointment of education directors in an increasing number of NHS regions, with a co-ordinating role right across these funding streams which are of such central importance to 'human resource development', provides the opportunity to enhance positive interaction between these funding streams.

Complexity of regulatory arrangements

The existence of different statutory bodies for regulation of medicine, nursing, midwifery and different PAMs, while not a constraint to the development of interprofessionalism per se, certainly complicates its management.

Table 12.2 Main funding streams involved in education and research associated with the NHS

HEFCE:	Higher Education Funding Council for England (an 'arm's length' agency of the Department of Education and Employment).
SIFT:	Service increment for teaching (an NHS levy funded by the Department of Health to meet clinical service facility and placement costs of undergraduate medical and dental education).
R&D:	Various research-related NHS budgets funded by the Department of Health to meet the costs of NHS research and the NHS service costs of other agencies' research.
MRC:	Medical Research Council.
AMRC:	Association of Medical Research Charities.
MADEL:	Medical and Dental Education levy of the NHS to meet the costs of postgraduate medical and dental education in the NHS.
NMET:	Non-medical education training levy.

Conclusions

Several current trends will encourage a productive relationship between universities and their local HImPs, not least of which is the general geographical location of medical and health science schools in or close to areas where health improvement is most needed. The reforms in MB BS education following *Tomorrow's Doctors*[(6)], the lead role of academic general practice and, to a lesser extent, academic public health in many schools, and the excellent research opportunities developing in the primary care field are all encouraging greater medical school support for local health improvement.

On the other hand, poor recruitment to nursing generally, and of doctors to general practice, the dominance of short-term pressures in clinical service, the load of RAE, TQA and clinical governance on academic staff and others involved in teaching staff are damaging. The lack of a major clinically active academic workforce in nursing also appears to be a major shortcoming, although the increasing opportunity to develop the interprofessional agenda positively helps balance this. Perhaps the greatest threat is an unrealistic short-term expectation of HImPs, leading to unsustainable pressures on the relatively limited workforce of clinical academic leaders able to work across the school-HImP divide.

Health improvement is a long-term issue and the track record has not been too bad. Since Florence Nightingale's *Notes on Nursing* (see quote on page 85) was published with its modern perspective on multifactorial causation, intergenerational effects and primary and community care, a steady improvement in life expectancy, minimization of disease burden and enhancement of life for those with disability has been observed. Much more remains to be done, but if the next generation can continue the trajectory of improvement seen over the past 150 years and increasingly focus on the most deprived areas this will, in itself, be a considerable achievement.

Key messages

- Medical and health service schools are often located in deprived areas
- Mutual support between the NHS and universities is essential if either is to thrive
- The ability at local level to mount a successful HImP depends critically on the locality's ability to recruit and retain able staff
- The role of medical schools is not limited to education, research and provision of clinical services and includes the direct contribution to the local wider community
- The greatest threat to HImP is unrealistic short-term expectations leading to unsustainable pressures on the relatively limited workforce working across the academic-service divide
- Knowledge and scholarship based on research is essential for effective interventions to improve health.

Acknowledgement

I am extremely grateful to many colleagues, especially Professors Sean Hilton and Mike Pittilo, for their inspiring and vigorous approach to these issues. The mistakes and errors of emphasis in this very personal view are, of course, my own.

References

1 Richards R. *Clinical academic careers*. Report commissioned by the Committee of Vice-Chancellors and Principals. London: CVCP, 1997.

2 McNicoll IH. *The impact of the universities and colleges on the UK economy*. London: Committee of Vice-Chancellors and Principals, University of Strathclyde, 1997.

3 Glenarthur, Lord. *Hansard* 1997, 25th February.

4 Steering Group on Undergraduate Medical and Dental Education (SGUMDER). *Ten key principles*. 4th report of SGUMDER. London: Department of Health and Department of Education and Employment, 1996.

5 NHS Executive, Committee of Vice-Chancellors. *Joint declaration of principles: nursing, midwifery and professions allied to medicine. Contracts for education and training with institutions of higher education in England*. Leeds: NHS Executive and CVCP, 1998.

6 General Medical Council (UK). *Tomorrow's doctors, recommendations on undergraduate medical education*. London: GMC, 1993.

7 Dobson F. *Hansard* 1999: 11th January.

8 Foskett NH, Hemsley-Brown JV. *Perceptions of nursing as a career*. Southampton: Centre for Research and Education Marketing, University of Southampton, 1998.

9 Boyd R. *International performance of UK medical institutions*. *Lancet* 1997; **350**: 595–6.

►13

New therapies and technology

Mr Norman Evans
Pharmaceutical Advisor, Merton, Sutton and Wandsworth Health Authority, London, UK

Dr Stuart Atkinson
Principal Medical Advisor, Pfizer Limited, London, UK

The last quarter of this century must be the most technically advanced in human history and many more advances are to come as we enter the millennium. Technology has had a huge impact on the ways in which healthcare is delivered and human disease is treated. Advances in molecular genetics and the microchip mean that many diseases today can be diagnosed accurately and targeted with specific treatment. While the benefits are obvious, the costs and risks are often not fully assessed, yet such technologies enter the NHS at a speed many health planners and policy makers find difficult to cope with.

Managing the entry of new therapies and technologies into the NHS, therefore, is a challenging process likely to have a significant financial and clinical impact. Using new drugs, for example, may expose patients to unforeseen risks, while delays in use might deny them benefit. The difficulty for commissioners and providers of healthcare is that, while new technologies might confer distinct advantages over existing therapies, at the time of introduction there is often insufficient good quality evidence to define their place in therapy. This can result in the slow uptake of beneficial innovations, variations in interpretation of data resulting in variable uptake across the country and a waste of resources when treatments are not used in their most cost-effective manner.

The challenge for the NHS is the early identification, assessment and appraisal of new technologies so that their introduction can be planned to give maximum benefit and value for money[(1)].

Identification of new technologies

The need for evidence-based forecasting in healthcare is essential to avoid the haphazard introduction of new technologies before full evaluation has taken place. Beneficial technologies need to be introduced in a planned way and the early detection of innovations likely to have an impact on the health economy is important. This will become increasingly so with current changes in the delivery of healthcare in the UK.

With the devolution of commissioning power to primary care groups (PCGs) it will become imperative to ensure equity of access to advances shown to provide health gain. Attempts to plan or halt the diffusion of technological innovations have been unsuccessful[(2)]. To resolve this problem the National Horizon Scanning Centre (NHSC) has been established at the University of Birmingham[(3)]. This will seek to identify to the Department of Health new and emerging health technologies at the

Table 13.1 Identification of new technologies

- Local, national and international networks
- Licensing agencies
- Development and manufacturing companies
- News and financial media

Table 13.2 Scope of National Horizon Scanning Centre (NHSC)

- Pharmaceuticals
- Devices
- Diagnostic tests and procedures
- Interventional devices
- Rehabilitation and therapy
- Service delivery and organizational topics

earliest opportunity (Table 13.1). It will work in close collaboration with other organizations such as the National Prescribing Centre, UK Drug Information Pharmacists Group, National Co-ordinating Centre for Health Technology Assessment (NCCHTA) and Euro-Scan (European Information Network on New and Changing Health Technologies). It will use expert judgement to assess the potential significance of its funding to the NHS (Table 13.2).

The objective is to identify new technologies that require further evaluation, consideration of clinical and cost-effectiveness or the development of clinical guidance. Once identified, a process of prioritization will be used to discard trivial changes and additional information sought for the most significant advances. Anyone encountering a new or emerging technology is invited to send any relevant information to the NHSC (0121 414 7582).

Evaluation

Having identified and prioritized new developments, the NHSC will pass the information on to other bodies, notably the National Institute of Clinical Excellence (NICE), established in April 1999. This will be the principal organization for developing evidence-based guidelines for nationwide use. There are, however, many other organizations involved in the evaluation of new health technologies (Table 13.3).

NICE will, however, probably be the main vehicle for providing guidance on new innovations and the appraisal of existing interventions. It will regularly examine all interventions likely to be introduced into the NHS. Its scope will be similar to the NHSC and include population-screening procedures. The appraisal process within NICE will be carried out by a multiprofessional group and advice then issued direct to the NHS. It is intended that the work will be available before the launch of any intervention.

Table 13.3 UK network organizations evaluating health technologies

- National Prescribing Centre
- UK Drug Information Pharmacists Group
- Safety and Efficacy Register of New Interventions and Procedures
- Regional Developmental and Evaluation Committees
- National Co-ordinating Centre for Health Technology Assessment
- Medical Devices Agency
- Standing Medical Advisory Committee
- MRC and other research councils
- UK Focus for Biomedical Engineering
- Office of Science and Technology
- NHS Centre for Reviews and Dissemination
- Department of Health-sponsored groups and programmes

Introduction and implementation

It is to be presumed that the guidelines produced by NICE will be implemented locally into the NHS but there will obviously be a transition period until the organization reaches maturity in about three years' time. During this period health authorities will still be charged with managing the introduction of new technologies into the NHS according to HSG(94)72. Under this directive, most health authorities have established committees to manage the introduction of drugs and appliances locally. They have decided whether or not products should be used and if so whether in secondary, primary or shared care, between consultants and GPs[(4)].

A scheme for evaluating and introducing new products in Merton, Sutton and Wandsworth Health Authority is shown in Figure 13.1. Its prescribing committee has representatives from primary and secondary care and patient groups. An early decision, which has proved useful, was not to recommend a product within six months of launch in order to allow as full an evaluation as possible to take place. Lists have been drawn up of products which should only be prescribed by consultants and those which can be prescribed under shared-care agreements. The committee also considers new indications for licensed products.

The recent Government white paper *The New NHS*[(5)] has proposed many changes to the strategic and operational directions of the NHS (PCGs, health improvement programmes and clinical governance). These will take time to develop and until NICE is fully operational it will be vital to ensure fairness between practices and patients in getting the treatment and resources they clinically need. Meanwhile, accepting that it is very difficult and in most circumstances impossible to resist the entry of new technology and therapy to the NHS, the following questions have to be addressed sensitively and through partnership with other health organizations:

- What is the magnitude of health improvement attributable to the new technology?
- How should the cost of new technology/therapy be met? (invest)
- Is the new therapy/technology a replacement for the old? (de-invest)
- Can savings be identified outside the NHS (social services, etc)?

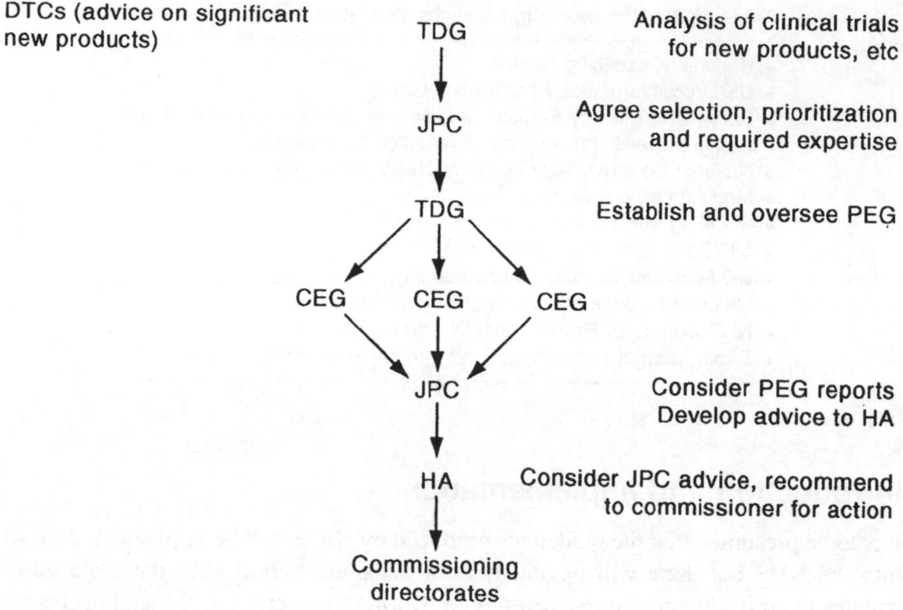

Fig. 13.1 Scheme for evaluating and introducing new products.
TDG = therapeutic development group, JPC = joint prescribing committee, CEG = clinical effectiveness group, HA = health authority, DTC = drugs and therapeutic committee.

- For new frontiers (new needs) with limited resources, who should determine priorities?
- How should patients/the public be involved with the decisions to introduce new technology and made fully aware of the benefits, risks and costs (NHS, social, personal, etc)?

The key question on the mind of every clinician and policy maker is 'is it ethical to recommend new therapy and raise patients' expectations for better health and better life if the money is not available?'

Conclusions

The granting of a product licence or marketing authorization by the European Medicines Evaluation Authority is unlikely to guarantee a product's acceptance by the NHS. New technologies will be subject to further scrutiny by various bodies and recommendations and guidelines issued. It is to be hoped that this will mean faster uptake of beneficial innovations and more effective use of resources through the elimination of interventions shown to be of no value. The dilemma is how to balance the introduction of needed and effective interventions on the one hand with their costs on the other.

Key messages

- Technological advances have made a significant contribution to many innovative healthcare interventions
- Innovations will enable more conditions to be treated (needs) and increase patients' expectations (demands)
- It is difficult to resist the introduction of new technology but at what cost does this happen and how should costs be met?
- The public should be fully involved with the introduction of new technology and made aware of the benefits, risks and costs.

References

1 Simister KL, Jackson CW. Informing the effective introduction of drugs into the NHS. *Pharmaceutical J* 1998; **261**: 90–2.
2 Doyle YG. New medical technologies. *Ir Med J* 1996; **90**: 50–1.
3 National Prescribing Centre. *Connect* 1998; **14**.
4 Wakeman A, Leach R. Joint prescribing committee: characteristics, progress and effectiveness. *Health Trends* 1997; **29**: 52–4.
5 Secretary of State for Health. *The new NHS: modern and dependable*. London: The Stationery Office, 1997.

▶14

Coronary heart disease: a practical tool and structured approach to developing and implementing a HImP

Dr Nicholas R Hicks
Consultant in Public Health Medicine, Oxfordshire Health Authority, UK

Dr Rachel Crowther
Specialist Registrar, Oxfordshire Health Authority, UK

One of the main aims of this book is to highlight, through expert discussion, the best pathways along which to develop and implement health improvement programmes (HImPs) at the local level, balancing national and local priorities. In this chapter we share a real-life example of work being undertaken in the NHS to develop a practical tool to help those charged with developing and implementing HImPs. The example describes 'work in progress', 'warts and all'. While we have not managed to provide a miracle tool for those faced with HImP development, our shared experiences may help others to frame their thinking on the subject and to offer us useful criticism and advice.

Collaborative brief to develop a coronary heart disease HImP

In the spring of 1998, the Directors of Public Health for the nine health authorities of the old Oxford and Anglia Region (covering a population of about five million) asked one of us (NH) to work with nominated representatives from each of these counties to develop a practical approach for producing a HImP. We were asked to illustrate our approach with coronary heart disease (CHD) for the following reasons:

- CHD is a national priority for which an early national service framework is being developed
- CHD is a local priority for many health authorities
- Oxfordshire had recently won the Health Services Management Award for its involvement in the NHS Executive/Conference of Royal Colleges pilot project on the Care Programme Approach to CHD
- Social class inequalities in CHD mortality rates have tripled between the 1970s and 1990s
- 'Broad determinants' of health and clinical practice are both important influences on CHD morbidity and mortality.

In most cases the representatives from each county were also the CHD leads for their county.

Aims

We began by reminding ourselves that the white paper *The New NHS*[(1)] and subsequent guidance (including *Partnerships in Action*) set out the following expectations for HImPs:

- to set the *strategic direction* for
  - improving health
  - reducing inequalities
  - delivering more integrated, user-centred health and social care
- to set the *framework for action* on health and for commissioning services
- to set *targets and milestones* for achieving measurable improvements.

HImPs are expected to become the framework for local health strategy and a focus in which health authorities, local authorities and other partners could work together to 'identify how local action on social, environmental and economic issues will make most impact on the health of the local people'[(1)].

Together with the commitment to high-quality clinical care set out in *A First Class Service*[(2)], the emphasis on local partnerships and practical solutions forms a cornerstone of the Government's new approach to the NHS. However, translating the concept of a HImP into a programme of work is a complex and challenging process for health authorities and their local partners. We will all make mistakes—there is much to be gained from sharing practical experience.

Success criteria

It was agreed at the outset that certain criteria must be met if the group's work was to be successful. The tool developed had to be:

- *practical*, supporting the implementation and not just the development of the HImP on paper
- *focused on health* and the determinants of health as well as healthcare
- *multisectorial*—relevant and usable by different agencies
- *quantifiable* in terms of outcomes
- *understandable* to the general public.

Developing the tool

The group was keen to relate its work clearly to Government policy. It therefore took its starting point as *The New NHS*[(1)] and *Our Healthier Nation*[(3)], in particular the National Contract on Heart Disease from *Our Healthier Nation* which sets out the responsibilities and action to be taken by different groups—individuals, local players and communities, Government and national players. The contract for health classifies the range of determinants of health into four groups:

- social and economic
- environmental

- lifestyle
- services.

In the vocabulary of the National Contract, health authorities and local authorities are 'local players'.

The group decided to look at ways of developing the community and hospital service (CHS) section of the HImP that mapped to the 'local players and communities' column of the National Contract for Health. It rapidly became apparent that no matter which determinant of cardiac health we discussed—housing or aspirin, physical activity or cardiac rehabilitation, smoking or employment—similar sets of questions were asked. For example, for every topic: we wanted to know how important a determinant of cardiac health it was, what were the possible means of intervening, and was there any evidence about the effectiveness of intervention. Similarly, in thinking about implementation, we wanted to agree the relative priority of a particular action, to identify the organization that would be responsible for leading action, the resources to be deployed and other similar practical issues.

We compiled a grid consisting of a list of the questions which we thought might be relevant to any topic that was to be included in a HImP (Table 14.1). The intention was that the rows of the grid should reflect our questions and the columns should refer to particular determinants of health such as exercise, smoking or coronary revascularization procedures. Essentially, the grid acts as a prompt and checklist of those questions which people should ask about determinants of health and potential interventions, but often do not: it represents a straightforward, but systematic, approach to decision-making and the development of HImPs. This was our proposed tool to help in the production and implementation of HImPs.

Table 14.1 HImP development and implementation grid

Topic (eg) smoking
Why is it relevant to health?
What is the evidence that it is relevant?
Where are we now? (local/national baseline)
What are the relevant factors or characteristics of the local population?
What is the cost of current provision?
What action/intervention is needed?
What is the evidence on effectiveness of this action?
Who needs to act?
What is the expected health impact?
What resources are needed?
Who will pay?
What level of priority should it have?
Who will benefit?
What are the barriers or obstacles to achieving change?
What opportunities are there for linking with national guidance (for health or other agencies)?
What are the key targets?
What are the milestones/dates?
What are the monitoring criteria?
Who will monitor?
How will action be communicated and to whom?

Preliminary piloting

We wanted to know whether the grid (the tool) would be of practical use to those developing HImPs and whether it would work for both clinical and non-clinical determinants of health. Each member of the nine-county group volunteered to use the grid to 'work up' a different determinant of cardiac health in their county, eg smoking, housing, employment and coronary revascularization.

This stage of the project has generated uncharacteristic enthusiasm and energy. Everyone reported that they had been surprised at how easy it was to use the grids and how useful the process of completing the grid had been. The grids allowed information on complex issues to be organized and presented in a straightforward and consistent way and facilitated productive and practical debate with other agencies. The grids had already catalysed many useful local discussions, which had led to ideas about potential topics for local collaboration and new ways of working together. For example:

- Counties identified previously untackled determinants of health, eg the group working up housing was surprised at the magnitude of excess winter mortality from CHD in the UK that was not found in the colder climates of Scandinavia (Table 14.2).
- Other counties identified new ways of sharing data, monitoring the impact of local policies and measuring local inequalities, eg the group working up employment identified non-NHS data that they recommended be published regularly in the local Director of Public Health's Annual Report (Table 14.3).

Table 14.2 Grid for housing and CHD

Why is it relevant to health?	Cardiovascular changes increase the risk of myocardial infarction and stroke when room temperature falls below 12°C[(1)]
What is the evidence that is relevant?	Excess mortality in winter: about 40,000 more people die in Britain in winter than in summer; most are older people Excess deaths are mostly due to respiratory and cardiovascular diseases, not hypothermia Report of the Building Research Establishment[(1)] concluded that defining a safe lower limit for house temperatures was impossible but that risk to health increases as temperature falls
What action/intervention is needed?	Standards should be set so that an acceptable indoor temperature, say 20°C, can be achieved at no more than 10% of the household income. Any excess needed should be provided in social payments[(2)]
Who will benefit?	The poorest in society: the unemployed, the chronically sick, older people[(2)] 'Fuel poverty' describes those with least to spend on heating but living in houses that are hard to heat. Many low-cost houses are prone to cold and damp[(2)]
What are the key targets?	Indoor temperature of local authority housing stock to be kept at a minimum of 20°C

Table 14.3 Grid for Employment and CHD

What are the monitoring criteria? who will monitor?	*Labour force survey:* This is a continuous survey of a sample of 120,000 individuals in 61,000 households in any three-month period. The survey uses the International Labour Organization definition of unemployment and includes all people who are unemployed and seeking work. It covers men aged 16–64 and women aged 16–59. Since April 1998, results have been published 12 times a year, each covering the average for a three-month period and each available six weeks after the period they refer to. These data are useful for international and regional comparisons and provide a more complete picture of unemployment, especially in women. The results are produced by the Socio-Economic, Statistics and Analysis Group of the Office of National Statistics (ONS). *Claimant count:* number of people claiming unemployment-related benefits on a particular day each month. Results are published five weeks after the period they refer to and are available at ward level. These data are more useful for subregional comparisons and provide a timely indicator of recent changes in employment. They are provided by the employment service; small area statistics are available from NOMIS (Tel: 0191 3742468).

Advantages and problems

In general, the group identified the strengths and weaknesses of using the grid. Potential *advantages* included:

- general HImP development:
  - enables a range of partner agencies and organizations to be engaged in the debate around the HImP
  - promotes constructive dialogue focused on practical local issues
  - can be used equally effectively to look at diverse determinants of health (from education to smoking or housing to exercise—and for healthcare services, too)
  - supports both the social and medical 'models' of health
  - helps to identify issues that must be considered locally, such as the practicalities of local implementation, or the need for local debate about relative priorities, and distinguishes them from the following issues
  - reveals issues that could be considered nationally or regionally, eg areas where legislation may be desirable or more evidence is needed to support decision-making.
- decision-making:
  - promotes the consideration of valid, relevant evidence as one 'brick' in the process
  - facilitates comparison and priority setting across programmes by allowing different issues to be placed side by side.
- implementation:
  - links strategy and planning
  - specifies the interventions that are needed and are practical

- allows clear targets to be set and progress measures to be identified
- specifies who should take responsibility for particular areas.

Potential *problems* included:

- general points:
  - some topics are too 'large' for the grid and require segmentation and greater focus
  - work required to complete some of the cells of the grid is substantial. However, those cells that do not require locality-specific data need to be completed only once for the country as a whole
  - broader determinants of health (eg employment, housing, transport) do not lend themselves to a disease-specific approach
  - focusing a debate on effects and outcomes reveals different players' values, which are sometimes uncomfortable and difficult to manage
  - grid exposes gaps in local organizations' information base and managerial decision-making structures and processes
  - grid supports a care-programme approach, which institutions are not yet organized to implement or manage
- specific points:
  - there is insufficient information during the first year of a HImP for the grid to be useful at this stage: CHD sections will tend to contain only 'headlines'. The grid is likely to be of greater use in future years.

What needs to happen next

Once the HImPs have been developed to the stage at which detailed negotiation and planning take place, we hope to undertake a more formal pilot of the grid involving all key stakeholders, including health authorities, primary care groups, local government, NHS trusts and other local partners. It is anticipated that the grid may be used in a variety of ways:

- Starting point to the HImP process to stimulate discussion with partner agencies, although not necessarily following the questions set out in the grid
- Basis for the planning process using the questions set out in the grid as a 'checklist' of areas for discussion
- Basis for the final structure of the HImP, recording what has been agreed by filling in the boxes in the grid
- 'Hypertext' for the HImP, ie to provide the background of evidence and thinking which underpins the final document.

The grids can be supplied to local groups in various ways:

- Blank grid, just showing the questions to be addressed.
- Sets of grids covering key topics for a HImP for CHD, such as smoking, secondary prevention and other areas suggested by the National Contract on Heart Disease in *Our Healthier Nation*, including transport and education, in which the cells for evidence have been completed to provide a basis for discussion and debate.

- Examples of completed grids produced by members of the nine-county CHD-HImP group for the same topics, where most of the cells have been filled in with suggested answers to the questions.

Before the formal pilot gets underway, the 'evidence' sections should ideally be completed rigorously and systematically so that the quality of information they contain is high. This is an example of the kind of task that could usefully be undertaken nationally, with regular updating to ensure that HImP development is based on up-to-date evidence of effectiveness and cost-effectiveness.

Conclusions

The provisional conclusions we can draw are that:

- The grid is a tool that can be used to help develop and implement HImPs
- A structured approach to developing and implementing HImPs may improve the quality of debate between local players, local decisions and management of implementation
- The tasks that need to be undertaken locally (eg local priority and target setting, agreeing specific organizational and individual responsibilities and allocation of local resources) can be distinguished from those that might more efficiently be undertaken nationally, eg reviewing evidence of effectiveness and cost-effectiveness of intervention
- The grid has helped to identify some of the roles that the Department of Health might play in supporting local players as they develop and implement HImPs: commending a structured and systematic approach to HImP development and implementation; providing information on the contribution of different determinants of health and of the evidence of the effectiveness and cost-effectiveness of different approaches to intervention.

Key messages

- Translating the concept of a HImP into a programme of work is a complex process for health authorities and local partners
- There is much to be gained from sharing practical experience
- Success criteria for any HImP are practicable, focused on health, multisectorial, quantifiable and understandable to the general public
- It is necessary to develop the appropriate tools to help to develop and implement a HImP
- A structured approach is also necessary for the development and implementation of a HImP.

Acknowledgement

We thank Professor Raj Bhopal for his helpful comments and advice. This work was undertaken on behalf of the Anglia and Oxford Nine Counties Coronary Heart Disease Health Improvement Programme Group.

References

1 Secretary of State for Health. *The new NHS: modern and dependable*. London: The Stationery Office, 1997.
2 Department of Health. *A first class service: quality in the new NHS*. London: DoH, 1998.
3 Secretary of State for Health. *Our healthier nation: a contract for health*. A consultative document. London: The Stationery Office, 1998.

▶15

Equity in mental health

Professor Rachel Jenkins
Director of Psychiatry, WHO Collaborating Centre, Institute of Psychiatry, London, UK

Dr Geraldine Strathdee
Consultant Psychiatrist, Institute of Psychiatry, London, UK

Ms Sarah Carr
Research and Information Officer, The Implemens Network, London, UK

Dr Salman Rawaf
Director of Clinical Standards/Senior Lecturer, Merton, Sutton and Wandsworth Health Authority, London, UK

There are substantial inequalities in the distribution of mental illness, in services for people with mental illness and in the outcomes achieved by those services. Health improvement programmes (HImPs) are being introduced to tackle such inequity. This paper aims to assist those working to establish the mental health aspects of a HImP.

HImP: policy framework

The policy framework for mental health is highlighted in many recent key strategic and operational documents on the reorganization and modernization of the NHS in Britain.

- The white paper, *The New NHS: Modern and Dependable*, outlines areas of action to improve national standards and develop guidelines to make the NHS a more 'modern, dependable' body[(1)]. Evidence-based national service frameworks are planned to help ensure consistent access to services and quality of care across the country. A National Institute for Clinical Excellence (NICE) is to give a strong lead on clinical practice and cost-effectiveness.

  The delivery of healthcare is to be measured against new national standards and is a matter of local responsibility. Health authorities are to work with local authorities, NHS trusts and primary care groups (PCGs) and take the lead in drafting three-year HImPs. HImPs will provide the framework in which all local NHS bodies will operate. Health authorities will allocate funds to PCGs on an equitable basis and hold them to account. A new Commission for Health Improvement is to support and oversee the quality of clinical services locally and tackle shortcomings[(1)].
- *Our Healthier Nation* proposes a drive to improve the health of the worst off in society and narrow the health gap[(2)]. It focuses on four priority areas with targets for improvement; one of these areas is mental health. A target has been set to reduce the death rate from suicide in 1996 by at least a sixth (17%) by 2010.

- Sir Donald Acheson's *Inequalities in Health Report*, the findings of which heavily inform *Our Healthier Nation*, recommends that: 'health authorities, working with primary care groups and providers on local clinical governance, agree priorities and objectives for reducing inequities in access to effective care. This should form part of the Health Improvement Programme'[3].

  Our Healthier Nation states that HImPs are to focus on particular health problems and health inequality, with scope to identify additional local priorities. Two suggested targets focus on environment (housing) and the needs of vulnerable groups (ethnic minorities, the homeless, people on low income and refugees)[2].
- *Modernising Mental Health Services*[4]. The plans to improve mental health services are to be a key part of HImPs, with 'modernization fund' targets to be developed for each HImP to establish a three-year plan which matches investments to measurable outcomes in service delivery. HImPs are to ensure that they make joint assessments of the mental health and social needs of the local population; audit current mental health service performance; identify gaps and pressures and develop joint investment plans to address them; and agree local priorities for action guided by the strategy document and local findings[4].

Evidence base for developing effective mental health services

Besides having information about the overall epidemiology of the various mental disorders and their relationship to sociodemographic variables, achieving effective mental health services depends on careful assessment of needs, attention to the range, quality and quantity of service inputs and processes and careful measurement of service outcomes in order to address inequities.

Mental health service user needs

Understanding the needs of people with severe mental illness is a fundamental step towards ensuring equity in mental health services and the development of services which lead to appropriate outcomes. Individuals with mental health disorders have a wide range of social and health needs, all of which concern issues of inequality and social exclusion. Research into the requirements of mental health service users has defined the following as priority areas of needs to be met[5,6]:

- appropriate housing and support
- enough money to live without hardship
- a meaningful day—leisure or work
- social and support networks
- physical and dental care
- medication and psychoeducation
- psychological treatments.

Carer needs

Over the past two decades, research has demonstrated that social and environmental factors play a major role in the development of disorders and in the prevention of relapse. This means that it is important to look after the needs of carers, not just for the sake of their own mental health, but also to reduce the risk of relapse in their relative.

Carers of people with mental illness, whether family or professional, also have needs that must be met if the mental health of their charge is to be improved and their vast contribution to care recognized. Most are concerned with easy and direct access to mental health services, respite care and practical support with welfare benefits, finance and housing. Carers also report that they need information and education on disorders, treatments and available services available, including crisis services which are rapidly responsive and have a single point of access[5,7].

Effective service structures

Achieving improved outcomes for the mentally ill can only be achieved through social and health service provision. A *systems approach* is vital. Traditional psychiatric hospitals often provided the full range of social and work rehabilitation services as well as medical and other clinical care within the institution. Developing community services requires the co-operation and collaboration of local authority housing and social services departments, primary care agencies, special Community Mental Health Teams (CMHTs), the health authority and often the voluntary sector (which provides housing, care, welfare benefits advice, work and rehabilitation projects, information and user support agencies).

Community care has meant that service developers need to work across several agencies to develop the full range of services to meet the needs of patients. Mental health service structures must be informed by sound principles of service development. There is a general consensus that services must be:

- local and accessible
- flexible and comprehensive to address diverse needs
- consumer-orientated and empowering to ensure that client need is met and clients are supported in gaining maximum control over their lives.

Care should be designed to focus on the strengths and skills of the service user and encourage independence; it needs to be normalized and incorporated into natural community supports. Services should be racially and culturally appropriate, with attention given to groups with special needs such as the homeless and those with physical disabilities. Service evaluation and accountability to the consumers and carers will ensure the continuing appropriateness and effectiveness of the care provided[8].

Accordingly, a comprehensive community mental health service needs to integrate a series of structures and components. Systematically and jointly assessed local and population needs identification must inform strategic and operational plans.

Although there has been a great deal of debate as to what constitutes an effective service structure in mental health services, there is little consensus about what constitutes an effective service relevant to each local area. Most of the work has been policy rather than research driven (national service frameworks, Clinical Standards Adivisory Group [CSAG] on schizophrenia, Health Advisory Service [HAS], etc). The uniquely consistent finding is that for individuals with severe and enduring mental illnesses an *assertive community treatment* (ACT) approach is needed[9]. A recent

Cochrane international research review concluded that: 'ACT is an effective alternative to standard care and to hospital-based rehabilitation in patients with severe mental disorders'[10].

The key features of an effective assertive outreach team include[11,12]:

- delivery by a multidisciplinary team, usually including a psychiatrist, nurse and at least two case managers
- low staff: client ratios (1 : 10)
- most services provided in the community (in people's homes or cafés) rather than in an office setting
- caseloads shared across clinicians rather than each having an individual caseload
- 24-hour coverage
- time-unlimited service
- most services directly provided by the ACT team and not brokered out.

One of the key challenges for local services is to agree how the necessary ACT services should be provided locally. In high morbidity inner-city areas, services are most likely to be successful if they are provided by a small, protected team. In low morbidity areas, CMHTs use a caseload, case-mix process whereby staff have between 60 and 80% of people with severe mental illness on their caseloads.

Acute inpatient beds are the most expensive resource and should therefore be used only for sound therapeutic reasons[8]. Evidence-based community alternatives to hospital admission include crisis response services such as acute home treatment teams[13–15] and day hospitals which can provide support, supervision and monitoring, as well as being sites for intensive therapy[16,17]. Twenty-four-hour nursed care is a small but crucial component for the small number of people who are so ill that they need 'round the clock' trained care and supervision, particularly in areas of high social deprivation with a large population of individuals living alone.

Effective interventions

Even if mental health service structures are improved, outcomes for users with severe mental illness will only improve where there is an analysis of existing staff skills and funding dedicated to training in new skills in order to enable the routine use of effective interventions[18]. The list below is not comprehensive but outlines some of the most important interventions, which are social as well as clinical:

- housing with adequate support
- welfare benefits and financial advice
- physical and dental care
- medication and psychoeducational programmes
- cognitive behavioural therapy for psychotic symptoms
- identification and development of coping strategies
- family and carer education, support and therapies
- crisis and relapse prevention
- rehabilitation, practical skills and support
- day care
- work and education.

Evidence to support the effective use of psychoeducation and cognitive behavioural therapy for people with severe mental illness is emerging[19,20]. Research reviews have suggested that psychoeducational interventions such as 'coping strategy enhancement' can help to reduce psychotic symptoms when used in conjunction with the appropriate medication[21]. Treatment adherence can also be improved among people with chronic psychotic illness using educational and medication management strategies[22]. A key need for local HImPs is to ensure that staff working in both mental health services and local supported housing schemes are trained in this effective range of interventions.

Measurable outcomes and clinical effectiveness and efficiency

Table 15.1 summarizes some of the range of user, carer and service outcomes, which can be measured and used to assess the provision of effective mental health services. The table is not exhaustive and there are ranges of standardized instruments which can be used for each of the areas suggested.

Thus, the effectiveness of mental health services can be assessed using a number of outcome measures. The progress of the service user in terms of clinical status and social functioning as well as improvement in quality of life yield useful outcome data[23,24]. Whether or not users are satisfied with the treatment and care received from individual staff and the service as a whole is also important. The levels of carer involvement, the extent of carer contribution to individual care planning and the levels of information received also need to be considered. In relation to the monitoring of service use, use of hospital and community services, caseloads and case mixes is

Table 15.1 Measurable outcomes in mental health

User outcomes:
clinical status: decrease in symptoms
social functioning
extent of social network
quality of life
user satisfaction with services
user increase in knowledge about conditions and treatments
percentage of met and unmet needs under the care programme approach (CPA)
Carer outcomes:
all entitled benefits
practical support and respite
decrease in own mental health morbidity
carer satisfaction with services
carer increase in knowledge about conditions, treatments and services
percentage of met and unmet needs under the Carer's Act (1995) assessments
Service use outcomes:
rate of engagement and missed contact
decrease in relapse
decrease in unplanned admissions
decrease in length of stay
decrease in emergency consultation to primary care
decrease in admissions under a Section of the Mental Health Act (1983)
increase in staff recruitment and retention
increase in staff morale

essential information. Staff morale, motivation and levels of burnout and sickness also indicate service effectiveness[25].

Effective services and interventions for specific client groups

The integrated and comprehensive approach provided through HImP to reduce the burden of mental disorders and provide quality, effective and accessible services is described for three of the following major disease groupings:

- schizophrenia (Table 15.2)
- affective psychosis (Table 15.3)
- common mental disorder, eg depression (Table 15.4)
- dementia
- child psychiatry
- forensic psychiatry
- learning disability
- substance abuse.

Local health improvement programme

To achieve equity as part of local HImPs, a three-to-five-year strategic needs assessment plan needs to be undertaken locally. Table 15.5 proposes such a plan. The fundamental principles are that needs assessment at both provider and purchaser level should be jointly undertaken.

Stage 1: Locality-level data

This stage is about the collation of data on sociodemographic profiles and patterns of service need within public health departments. The Jarman, York and MINI indices provide crude data to enable the PCG locality to compare its indices against other local areas and national norms.

Stage 2: Profiling local services

The local services which contribute to demand on mental healthcare include:

- range of supported accommodation, including group homes, probation and hostels for the homeless, children and adolescent homes, etc
- housing configurations to include estates
- forensic services
- refugees
- level of single-handed GPs, group practices and health centres.

Stage 3: Practice-level data

This stage is an attempt further to refine data collection and analysis at the level of the practices within the locality. This is essential as often practices geographically proximate and therefore with similar sociodemographic profiles at the locality level

Table 15.2 Health improvement template for schizophrenia

HImP objectives	Underlying mechanisms	Effective interventions	Helpful input indicators for HImPs	Helpful outcome indicators for HImPs
To reduce incidence	Aetiology roughly half genetic (lifetime risk is 10–15% with one affected parent and 35–40% with two affected parents) and half environmental	Access to simple genetic counselling on request	Availability of simple genetic counselling on request	Local first episode figures
To shorten illness	Symptoms respond to medication. Newer antipsychotics may shorten first-onset illness in young men	Care programme paying attention to health and social care needs and incorporating adequate medication	CPA availability of newer antipsychotic medication	Health of the Nation Outcome Scale (HONOS) ratings at Care Programme Approach (CPA) reviews
To reduce relapse rates	Relapse can be precipitated by high levels of expressed emotion in families Patients can learn to recognize their own early warning signs of relapse Continued medication reduces risk of relapse	Relapse rates can be reduced 25% by using family interventions, 25% by direct education of sufferers about the early warning signs of relapse and by adequate maintenance therapy	Availability and training of staff in relapse prevention Incorporation of relapse prevention into care programme	Local readmission rates
Can disability be reduced?	Disability is greatly aggravated by institutionalization and inactivity	Rehabilitation services and access to adequate employment opportunities	Availability of sufficient quantity and quality of rehabilitation services Availability of employment opportunities	Health of the Nation Outcome Scale (HONOS) ratings at CPA reviews
To reduce mortality	Suicide (10–15% kill themselves) and physical illness, especially cardiovascular and respiratory disease and malignancy	Suicide prevention needs to be multifactorial: better assessment and management of individuals at risk; audit to learn lessons for prevention; support to high-risk groups; reduce access to means; work with media to ensure responsible reporting	Availability of good practice guidelines for suicide risk assessment and management Availability of physical health promotion and physical healthcare to people with severe mental illness; audit all suicides; guidelines for media	Local suicide rates of schizophrenics Local SMRs of schizophrenics

Table 15.3 Health improvement template for affective psychosis

HImP objectives	Underlying mechanisms	Effective interventions	Helpful input indicators for HImPs	Helpful outcome indicators for HImPs
To reduce incidence	Aetiology at least partially genetic[26] Morbid risk in relatives varies with uni- and bi-polar illness, age of onset and responsiveness totreatment		Genetic counselling services within the framework of primary and secondary care Continuing education of primary-care team about risk and advantages of prophylactic drug therapy Adequate employment opportunities Care registers to facilitate action and communication by care teams	Prevalence figures from the local psychiatric services, register supplemented by local community research services Hospital first-admission rates Employment rates Prevalence of suicide in local patients
To shorten illness		Illness episodes can be shortened by effective treatments including haloperidol and lithium	Continuing education of primary care teams about risk and advantages of prophylactic drug therapy	HONOS scores at CPA reviews
To reduce relapse rates		Relapse rates can be reduced by maintenance therapy with lithium and by direct education about early warning signs of relapse	CPA and care registers to facilitate action and communication by care teams	Hospital readmission rates HONOS scores employment rates
Can disability be reduced?			Adequate employment opportunities Care registers to facilitate action and communication by care teams	
To reduce mortality			Continuing education of primary and secondary care teams about assessment of suicide Adequate primary and physical health monitoring	Prevalence of suicide in local patients

Table 15.4 Health improvement template for depression

HImP objectives	Underlying mechanisms	Effective interventions	Helpful input indicators for HImPs	Helpful outcome indicators for HImPs
To reduce incidence	Causes of non-psychotic depression are environmental rather than genetic[27,28] Some depression is secondary to physical disease, pain and disability and is helped by the prevention and treatment of physical disease, pain and disability (particularly loss of mobility and sensory function, eg[29]) Some cases of depression are precipitated by acute life events and can be prevented by crisis intervention and other systems of support[30] Some is precipitated by lack of social support and can be prevented by setting up systems for at-risk groups (eg isolated mothers of preschool children). Organizations such as CRUSE and NEWPIN, as well as adequate child and family psychiatric services, may all help		Adequate screening and treatment facilities in primary care for physical disease and disability, loss of morbidity and sensory function System for primary care teams to identify those in their practice populations who are particularly at risk, including older people, young, isolated mothers of preschool children, the disabled and informal carers of severely physically or mentally ill patients, and to screen regularly, either opportunistically or on home visits where appropriate Resource indices in primary care, listing sources of support for their practice population Counsellors, psychologists and social workers in primary healthcare 'Stress' programmes in local workplaces with good collaboration between industry and healthcare teams Adequate training in detection (and treatment where appropriate) of depression for primary care teams, social services and occupational health services Active research studies on the causes, consequences and care of depression, particularly in primary care	Community surveys General practice identification index Prevalence of suicide and parasuicide
To shorten illness	Depression responds to psychological interventions, especially cognitive therapy, and to antidepressant treatment	Availability of staff trained in assessment and management, especially in cognitive behaviour therapy	Counsellors, psychologists and social workers in primary healthcare 'Stress' programmes in local workplaces with good collaboration between industry and healthcare teams Adequate training in and use of good practice guidelines for detection and treatment of depression for primary care teams, social services and occupational health services	
To reduce relapse rates	Relapse rates can be reduced by maintenance therapy with antidepressants and by cognitive therapy	Availability of staff in primary care who can do simple CBT		General practice consultation figures
Can disability be reduced?	Disability can be reduced by employment opportunities			Practice unemployment figures
To reduce mortality	A small proportion of people with nonpsychotic depression kill themselves Risk of death from all causes including accidents is twice the norm in severe psychotic depression			Local suicide and parasuicide figures

Table 15.5 Stages of needs assessment

Stage 1:	Epidemiological and public health data for the PCG locality
Stage 2:	Profiling of all locality services which will have an impact on healthcare demands
Stage 3:	Practice data to identify the sociodemographic indices per practice
Stage 4:	Needs assessment: Establishment of shared care case registers between primary and secondary care for individuals with severe and enduring and moderate mental illnesses
Stage 5:	Service use data to re-profile local resources

may have very different profiles at the practice level[31]. The reasons for this include the practice GPs' interest in particular conditions and willingness to provide care to group homes and hostels for the mentally ill, older adults with dementia who require residential care and children and adolescent homes. The range of practice sources which impact on mental health service needs at both primary and secondary care level include:

- practice size and population
- aggregated patients' data including new patient interviews to include:
  - gender and ethnicity
  - housing
  - marital status
  - children at school, in trouble, dyslexic
  - patients in prison and probation
  - drug misuse
  - alcohol misuse
  - domestic violence
  - carer status
- repeat prescriptions for psychotropic medications
- presence of practice counsellors, sessional community psychiatric nurses (CPNs), social workers, welfare benefits advisers, psychologists and psychiatrists.

Stage 4: Needs assessment

There is often a myth that people with mental health disorders are a largely transient population. The opposite is more often the case, with the exception of a few inner-city areas which attract large populations of homeless and transients. In the main, at least 80% of the local population with severe mental illness (SMI) remains in a given area. The joint establishment of a case register between primary and secondary care is therefore not a difficult task and is crucial for the equitable distribution of resources. As stated above, even within two practice 100 yards apart in an area of identical Jarman indices, the level of practice morbidity for SMI patients may be vastly different. Table 15.6 illustrates how, within an inner-city area of approximately 2 mile radius, practices have very significant differences in morbidity levels. Most of these differences, which have been replicated in several other areas in the country, can be explained in terms of the residential homes taken on by the practices.

In establishing case registers, Table 15.7 indicates the range of data sources.

Table 15.6 Distribution of SMI between practices in an inner-city area

Practice	Number of GPs	Number of SMI
1	10	121
2	3	98
3	1	26
4	5	52
5	3	56

Table 15.7 Data sources in establishing joint specialist-primary care case registers of the local mentally ill

Mental health service contacts	**Primary care team contacts**
CPA, supervision register and S.117 records	Practice register diagnosis of psychosis
CPN case loads	Repeat psychotropic drug prescriptions
Outpatient	Frequent emergency and other consultations
Domiciliary visit records	Hostel/group home/sheltered residence populations
Depot clinic patients	CPN attendees and health visitor contacts
Mental Health Act	
Inpatient audit data	
Crisis attendees (eg A&E attendees)	
Forensic service attender including court diversion, probation, prison	
Voluntary sector and other agency contacts	**Local authority contacts**
Residents of supported accommodation	Area social worker caseloads
Individuals causing local beat officers concern	Care management recipients
Imprisoned and homeless people	Housing department clients causing concern
Probation officer caseloads	People in receipt of bus passes and DLA
Drop-in and other casual facility users	People receiving care packages including carer support
User groups	
Individuals presenting to churches in distress	

Stage 5: Needs assessment for rational service planning

Having identified individuals with SMI in the CMHT locality, the next step is the introduction of a system of needs assessment. The routine collection of a clinical data set and care planning assessment and review is vital and, when incorporated into the CMHT culture, has the following effects:

- ensures that services are developed based on the aggregated needs of patients
- informs the case for resources
- facilitates multiagency co-ordination of services planning and delivery
- is vital at a national level for the mental health agenda[32].

Despite the many standardized assessment instruments in mental health, remarkably few are used in routine clinical practice. This discrepancy may arise because, although many instruments are helpful in monitoring symptoms, they do not lead directly to the informed decision making of management plans. In general, any innovation which is seen as a time-consuming addition to, rather than an integral part of, routine clinical practice is unlikely to succeed.

Newer instruments are a first stage in combining research validity with practical application. These include the Health of the Nation Outcome Scales and the Camberwell Assessment of Need. In many areas the CPA documentation is starting to combine several functions to avoid time-consuming duplication for clinicians. Efficiently implemented by clinicians, it can:

- serve as the accurate record of the met and unmet needs of the service user
- detail the agreed interventions with timescales for implementation and responsibilities and role of team members
- highlight risk and relapse prevention strategies.

It can also replace writing time-consuming lengthy letters to GPs and other agencies and can easily be communicated to users, carers and GPs and other involved agencies in line with confidentiality policies.

Conclusions

The aim and content of HImPs should reflect the spirit implicit in the name, ie improvement of health. Thus, HImPs should focus on the achievement of health gain and should move from finished treatment episode and contract currency to outcomes-led currency. The achievement of improved outcomes in mental health will depend on:

- careful assessment of needs of those with mental illness
- an appreciation of the evidence-base for interventions for treatment, rehabilitation and prevention of mortality for people with mental illness
- attention to the range, quality and quantity of service inputs and processes to deliver mental health interventions to best effect
- continuing assessment of mental health outcomes and interventions.

Key messages

- Many national policies are explicit in addressing inequalities in mental health
- Achieving effective mental health services depends on careful assessment of needs, attention to range, quality and quantity of service inputs and process, and careful assessment of service outcomes
- Care should be designed to focus on the strength and skills of service users and encourage independence, normalized into natural community support
- Outcomes in mental health can only be improved where staff skills are improved to the highest possible standards
- HImPs should move away from finished treatment episode and contract currency to outcomes-led currency.

References

1 Secretary of State for Health. *The new NHS: modern and dependable*. London: The Stationery Office, 1997.

2 Secretary of State for Health. *Our healthier nation: a contract for health*. Consultative document. London: The Stationery Office, 1998.

3 Acheson D (Chairman). *Independent inquiry into inequalities in health report*. London: The Stationery Office, 1998.

4 Department of Health. *Modernising mental health services: safe, sound and supportive*. London: Department of Health, 1998.

5 Audit Commission. *Finding a place: A review of mental health services for adults*. London: The Stationery Office, 1994.

6 Mental Health Foundation. *Creating community care: report of the Mental Health Foundation inquiry into care for people with severe mental illness*. London: Mental Health Foundation, 1994.

7 Thompson K, Carr S. What carers and families want from mental health services. In: Thompson K, Strathdee G, Wood H, eds. *Mental health skills development workbook*. London: The Sainsbury Centre for Mental Health, 1997: 5–6.

8 Strathdee G, Thornicroft G. Core components of a comprehensive mental health service. In: Thornicroft G, Strathdee G, eds. *Commissioning mental health services*. London: The Stationery Office, 1996: 133–45.

9 Wood H, Carr S. Designing local mental health services. In: Wood H, Carr S, eds. *Locality services in mental health: developing home treatment and assertive outreach*. London: The Sainsbury Centre for Mental Health/Northern Birmingham Mental Health NHS Trust, 1998.

10 Marshall M, Lockwood A. Review: assertive community treatment is an effective alternative in severe mental disorders. *Evidence-Based Mental Health* 1998; **1**(4):115.

11 Mueser K, Bond G, Drake R, Resnick S. Models of community care for severe mental illness: a review of research on case management. *Schizophr Bull* 1998; **24**(1): 37–74.

12 Sainsbury Centre for Mental Health. *The keys to engagement: review of care for people with severe mental illness who are hard to engage with services*. London: The Sainsbury Centre for Mental Health, 1998.

13 Hoult J. Community care of the acutely mentally ill. *Br J Psychiatry* 1986; **149**: 137–44.

14 Muijen M, Marks I, Connolly J *et al.* Home-based care and standard hospital care for patients with severe mental illness: a randomised controlled trial. *Br Med J* 1992; **304**: 749–54.

15 Burns T, Beadsmoore A, Bhat A *et al.* A controlled trial of home-based acute psychiatric services I: Clinical and social outcome. *Br J Psychiatry* 1993; **163** 49–54.

16 Sledge W, Tebes J, Rackfeld T. Acute respite crisis care. In: Phelan M, Strathdee G, Thornicroft G, eds. *Emergency mental health services in the community*. Cambridge: Cambridge University Press, 1995: 233–58.

17 Creed F, Black D, Anthony P *et al.* Randomised controlled trial of day versus inpatient psychiatric treatment *Br Med J* 1990; **300**: 1033–7.

18 Conway M, Shepherd G, Meltzer D. Effectiveness of intervention for mental illness and implications for commissioning. In: Thornicroft G, Strathdee G, eds. *Commissioning mental health services*. London: The Stationery Office, 1996: 247–64.

19 Kuipers E, Garety P, Fowler D *et al.* London-East Anglia randomised controlled trial of cognitive behavioural therapy for psychosis. I: effects of the treatment phase. *Br J Psychiatry* 1997; **171**: 319–27.

20 Kuipers E, Garety P, Fowler D *et al.* London-East Anglia randomised controlled trial of cognitive behavioural therapy for psychosis. II: predictors of outcome. *Br J Psychiatry* 1997; **171**: 420–6.

21 Penn D, Mueser K. Research update on the psychosocial treatment of schizophrenia. *Am J Psychiatry* 1996; **153**: 607–17.

22 Sair A, Bhui K, Haq S, Strathdee G. Improving treatment adherence among patients with chronic psychoses. *Psychiatric Bull* 1998; **22**: 77–81.

23 Department of Health. *The health of the nation key area handbook: mental illness*. 2nd ed. London: The Stationery Office, 1994.

24 Endicott J, Spitzler R, Fleiss J, Cohen J. The global assessment of functioning scale: a procedure for measuring overall severity of psychiatric disturbance. *Arch Gen Psychiatry* 1976; **33**: 766–71.

25 Strathdee G. The core components of comprehensive mental health services. In: Thompson K, Strathdee G, Wood H, eds. *Mental health skills development workbook*. London: The Sainsbury Centre for Mental Health, 1997.

26 Reich T, Claninger CR, Suarez B *et al.* Genetics of the affective psychoses. In: Wing JK, Wing L, Eds. *Handbook of Psychiatry. Volume 3. Psychoses of uncertain aetiology*. Cambridge: Cambridge University Press, 1982.

27 Torgensen S. Genetics of neuroses: the effects of sampling variation upon the twin concordance ratio. *Br J Psychiatry* 1983; **142**: 126–32.
28 Jenkins R. Minor psychiatric morbidity and labour turnover. *Br J Indust Med* 1985; **42**: 534–9.
29 Cooper AF. Deafness and psychiatric illness. *Br J Psychiatry* 1976; **129**: 216–26.
30 Newton J. Approaches to prevention: supporting troubled persons. In: *Preventing Mental Illness*. London: Routledge and Kegan Paul, 1988.
31 Strathdee G, Jenkins R, Carr S, Rawaf S. Equity in mental health—what public health practitioners should do. *Public Health Medicine* 1999; **2**: 61–7.
32 Kingdon D. The care programme approach. *Adv Psychiatric Treat* 1994; **1**: 41–4.

▶16

Substance misuse

Dr Salman Rawaf

Director of Clinical Standards/Senior Lecturer, Merton, Sutton and Wandsworth Health Authority, London, UK

Dr Owen Keyes-Evans

Senior Registrar in Public Health Medicine, Merton, Sutton and Wandsworth Health Authority, London, UK

Mrs Fiona Marshall

Specialist Nurse and Business Manager, Department of Addictive Behaviour and Psychological Medicine, St George's Hospital Medical School, London, UK

Professor Hamid Ghodse

Professor of Addictive Behaviour, St George's Hospital Medical School, London, UK

Scale of the problem

Substance misuse is widespread throughout society and has created different problems throughout the ages. Use and misuse of substances (prescribed and illicit drugs, over-the-counter (OTC) drugs, alcohol and nicotine) affects individuals, their families and society as a whole; there are no boundaries according to age, social class, race, religion, etc. Substance misuse is the cause of many social, behavioural, psychological and physical health problems[1,2]. There are high levels of comorbidity associated with substance misuse, both physical and psychological, and there are social and lifestyle consequences. There are also economic and international dimensions to the drug trafficking and organized crime aspects of the drug trade which add to the complexity of the picture and the need for local, national and international action.

While it is difficult to assess with accuracy, the prevalence of substance misuse appears to be rising, especially among young people and those in socially disadvantaged groups or otherwise excluded in some way. The Health Education Authority conducted two studies of young people, one in 1990[3,4] and one in 1995[5], and while not directly comparable, the trends indicated increasing experimentation. Substance use is still prevalent among more affluent groups, and although the associated problems of crime are not as damaging to society, individuals and families are still affected.

The national target areas outlined by the Department of Health in 1998 in the consultative document *Our Healthier Nation* are heart disease, cancer, accidents and mental illness[6]. Substance misuse affects all of these. The UK Anti-Drugs Co-ordinating Unit headed by a 'drug Tsar' and reporting directly to the cabinet has published a 10-year national strategy with four priority areas:

- young people
- treatment

- availability
- communities[7].

This national strategy depends on local action, co-ordinated by locally oriented drug action teams (DATs). Each DAT is developing its own action plan which is being assessed by the UK Anti- Drugs Co-ordinating Unit. A white paper on smoking was to be published in 1999 and a national strategy on alcohol is being developed. The Crime and Disorder Bill, Drug Treatment and Testing Orders and other community safety initiatives also address drug- and alcohol-related problems.

Substance misuse is therefore one of the main public health and social problems that modern societies face and has become a political priority (Table 16.1)

While the problems associated with drug use and misuse are many and complex, once individuals are dependent on certain substances the damage can be significant and permanent and interventions are often long term, involving many different agencies[8]. Effectiveness of treatment and interventions are measured in terms of stabilization, changes in lifestyle, employment and reduction in crime and harm to individuals as well as society (including improvements in quality of life). Most scientists and clinicians agree that addiction is a 'chronic relapsing condition'. Prevention, therefore, is the key strategic approach to tackling the problem of drug misuse and addiction[9].

Towards a HImP for substance misuse

The health improvement programme (HImP) is a reinvented policy concept in a modern and comprehensive format outlined in the white paper *The New NHS: Modern and Dependable*[10]. HImP is a local strategy for improving health and healthcare and reducing inequalities in health. It will be the means of delivering national targets in each health authority area, taking into account the local priorities and the burden of the problem in each locality. Key characteristics of a HImP are that:

- it is based on existing strategies
- there is full partnership with other agencies (particularly local authorities) in development and implementation
- the local health authority has lead accountability
- there are long- and short-term time-scales

Table 16.1 Current issues in substance misuse

Substance misuse:
- is public health problem number one
- will impact on future generations
- suffers rapidly changing trends
- has not just health, but social, political and economic dimensions
- is linked to other health issues
- has no single effective treatment against it
- suffers wide variation in clinical treatment
- suffers wide variation in service provision
- suffers policy confusion
- carries major scope for improvement

- there are measurable achievements in improving the health of the population or target group
- it can contribute to the development of measurable quality standards
- it is linked with service and financial frameworks
- there are supporting strategies.

The wide variety of substance use and misuse means that there is no single effective therapeutic response or lead agency. Interventions once dependence has been established are, in most cases, extremely complex. However, the key HImP development characteristics outlined above, particularly the need for partnerships and for existing strategies to be used, make substance misuse HImP development somewhat easier. DATs have already developed action plans and partnerships are already established and being further developed. DATs have development funding and joint commissioning arrangements are also being developed. The development of substance misuse HImPs provides an opportunity to strengthen DAT activity as well as feeding into local HImPs, improving health in all *Our Healthier Nation* target areas.

For the development of any HImP for substance misuse, a three-strand conceptual framework needs to be considered[9]:

- discouraging new recruits to drug and alcohol cultures and at least delaying the onset of use (*primary prevention*)
- discouraging continued use through treatment, contacting higher numbers of substance misusers and influencing their behaviour (*secondary prevention*)
- reducing the harm associated with misuse (*secondary and tertiary prevention*).

The comprehensive and integrated nature of such a framework provides a unique opportunity for working in partnership with many interested parties to mobilize community resources[9]. This model extends that proposed by the Advisory Council on the Misuse of Drugs[11] and the concept of reaching out to those not in contact with services is highlighted. Newer initiatives such as outreach services, arrest referral schemes, training initiatives for night club staff, etc have a significant role to play in such a model.

A variety of actions need to be taken to enact such a conceptual model: to be effective these need to be agreed at local levels. As discussed, there are a wide variety of national initiatives covering health, social services, the criminal justice system and providers of services. All these areas require the setting up of local multiagency groups/committees. There is a need to ensure that all these different groups reinforce each other, rather than compete or, at worst, obstruct. To develop a coherent HImP for substance misuse, the local DAT will need to be closely involved, but the health aspects need to be clearly defined so that lead agency status and outcome can be more clearly articulated and placed in the different local action plans. A useful approach could be to:

- define more accurately the various populations of interest which could be targeted by various agencies in collaboration and partnership
- increase knowledge and facilitate changes in attitude and behaviour, thus empowering individuals and communities to promote healthy environments and lifestyles

- influence clinical and organizational behaviour to redefine and reshape roles, functions, accountability and outcomes measurement.

Steps for HImP development

It is essential to develop a logistic and simple stepwise approach to achieve an appropriate and locally-sensitive HImP. Possible steps are described below.

Assessment

It is essential to form an accurate picture, as far as possible, of the prevalence and needs of the population and groups within the population. The assessment shoulc involve a degree of segmentation of the population in question to clarify the needs c different groups and subgroups (eg children need to be assessed according to differe age groups and subgroups, eg those in care or living in different areas of t community). Figure 16.1 illustrates an example of population segmentation and method of relating targets to each of the population groups in question[12].

Agencies working in partnership have to define the population of shared int and thus accept shared responsibility for achieving the specified targets. The vie different stakeholders will also assist in the development of the local picture. work such as local crime surveys will also help[13,14]. This process sho continued throughout the work as information on needs will assist in p measurement.

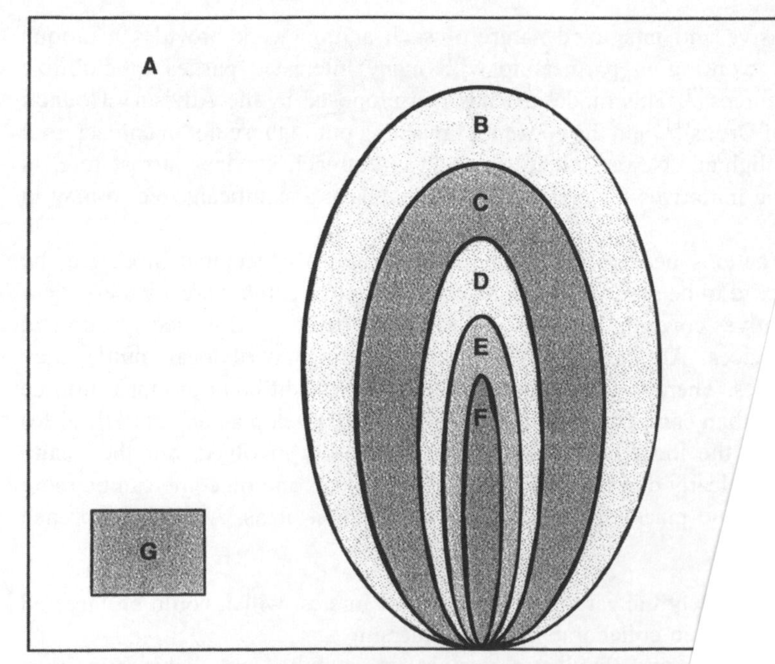

Fig. 16.1 Population segmentation with respect to drug use and misu
A = total population, *B* = parents, guardians and teachers, *C* = groups at high risk, *D* = experime... misusers, *F* = harmful use (addiction), *G* = prison population, *H* = special groups (eg pregnant women).

covered by all DATs such as smoking a should report to each DAT responsible fo be a mechanism to reconcile the statut enshrined under *The New NHS* legislation achieved by formal delegation of accounta However, as there are many different agen organizations relating to the DATs and ot HImPs are not often co-terminous, this may of primary care groups (PCGs) may ensure t remains at a health authority level, perhaps a public health will have a significant role monitoring health-related activity within the substance misuse-related HImP work.

Monitoring objective implementation

There must be a clear implementation stateme milestones, success measures and the methods the key responsible person. Organizations, s management and accountability systems as authority—democratic accountability to the ele central accountability to the NHS Executive; voluntary sector—to the founders and man monitoring a complex task.

Monitoring of health status

There will need to be clear outcome indicators to a HImP for substance misuse. Such outcome indic of[15]:

- individual outcomes (eg reduction in experimenta number of patients with long remission for more
- public health outcomes (eg reduction in the numb and hepatitis cases related to drug misuse, coron cases, alcohol-related admissions to A&E departr
- social outcomes (eg reduction in crime, family pr substance misuse) political indicators (eg increase positive reports on enforcement and street drug arrests and offences related to drugs)
- health indicators (eg reduction [or increase] in refe hospital, dual diagnosis, etc).

Service provision and clinical practice

There are wide variations both in service provision for d 16.2) and clinical practices in dealing with patients (Figu attributed to the variations in service provision, includi deal with substance misuse, lack of clear needs asses

- there are measurable achievements in improving the health of the population or target group
- it can contribute to the development of measurable quality standards
- it is linked with service and financial frameworks
- there are supporting strategies.

The wide variety of substance use and misuse means that there is no single effective therapeutic response or lead agency. Interventions once dependence has been established are, in most cases, extremely complex. However, the key HImP development characteristics outlined above, particularly the need for partnerships and for existing strategies to be used, make substance misuse HImP development somewhat easier. DATs have already developed action plans and partnerships are already established and being further developed. DATs have development funding and joint commissioning arrangements are also being developed. The development of substance misuse HImPs provides an opportunity to strengthen DAT activity as well as feeding into local HImPs, improving health in all *Our Healthier Nation* target areas.

For the development of any HImP for substance misuse, a three-strand conceptual framework needs to be considered[(9)]:

- discouraging new recruits to drug and alcohol cultures and at least delaying the onset of use (*primary prevention*)
- discouraging continued use through treatment, contacting higher numbers of substance misusers and influencing their behaviour (*secondary prevention*)
- reducing the harm associated with misuse (*secondary and tertiary prevention*).

The comprehensive and integrated nature of such a framework provides a unique opportunity for working in partnership with many interested parties to mobilize community resources[(9)]. This model extends that proposed by the Advisory Council on the Misuse of Drugs[(11)] and the concept of reaching out to those not in contact with services is highlighted. Newer initiatives such as outreach services, arrest referral schemes, training initiatives for night club staff, etc have a significant role to play in such a model.

A variety of actions need to be taken to enact such a conceptual model: to be effective these need to be agreed at local levels. As discussed, there are a wide variety of national initiatives covering health, social services, the criminal justice system and providers of services. All these areas require the setting up of local multiagency groups/committees. There is a need to ensure that all these different groups reinforce each other, rather than compete or, at worst, obstruct. To develop a coherent HImP for substance misuse, the local DAT will need to be closely involved, but the health aspects need to be clearly defined so that lead agency status and outcome can be more clearly articulated and placed in the different local action plans. A useful approach could be to:

- define more accurately the various populations of interest which could be targeted by various agencies in collaboration and partnership
- increase knowledge and facilitate changes in attitude and behaviour, thus empowering individuals and communities to promote healthy environments and lifestyles

- influence clinical and organizational behaviour to redefine and reshape roles, functions, accountability and outcomes measurement.

Steps for HImP development

It is essential to develop a logistic and simple stepwise approach to achieve an appropriate and locally-sensitive HImP. Possible steps are described below.

Assessment

It is essential to form an accurate picture, as far as possible, of the prevalence and needs of the population and groups within the population. The assessment should involve a degree of segmentation of the population in question to clarify the needs of different groups and subgroups (eg children need to be assessed according to different age groups and subgroups, eg those in care or living in different areas of the community). Figure 16.1 illustrates an example of population segmentation and the method of relating targets to each of the population groups in question[12].

Agencies working in partnership have to define the population of shared interest and thus accept shared responsibility for achieving the specified targets. The views of different stakeholders will also assist in the development of the local picture. Other work such as local crime surveys will also help[13,14]. This process should be continued throughout the work as information on needs will assist in progress measurement.

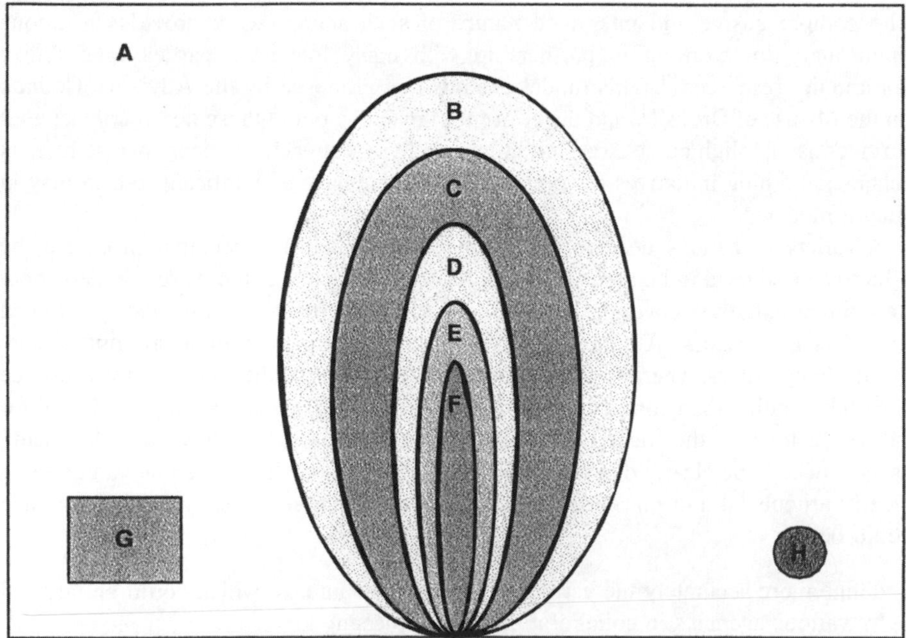

Fig. 16.1 Population segmentation with respect to drug use and misuse[12].
A = total population, *B* = parents, guardians and teachers, *C* = groups at high risk, *D* = experimenting and using drugs, *E* = drug misusers, *F* = harmful use (addiction), *G* = prison population, *H* = special groups (eg pregnant women).

Aim clarification

The aims of the substance misuse HImP should be clearly defined and agreed. They obviously need to be based on the results of the assessment and agreed by all involved in development of the HImP, including the DAT.

Objective or target setting

This step is essential and will also assist the group in further clarifying tasks. The objectives should specify what needs to be achieved in order to fulfil the aims of the HImP. They should be measurable and details given of how they are to be measured (ie quantify each of the objectives on a specific time-scale) and who should be the lead agency for each objective. This part of the HImP development should be intertwined with the DAT action plan, strengthening existing work, but also widening the scope to include alcohol and nicotine so that *Our Healthier Nation* target areas are addressed.

Definition of priorities for action and agreement of milestones

It must be recognized that a comprehensive programme to tackle the problem of substance misuse will involve multiple actions by many agencies at a variety of levels. With limited resources, both financial and human, it is essential to identify priorities and group them in terms of the effectiveness of the intervention to provide the maximum benefit in the shortest time. Milestones can be attached to the overall HImP but it may be helpful to define milestones for each of the objectives. This will assist in monitoring and evaluating success in a variety of dimensions.

Some actions could be achieved in the *short term* with no or little investment and may be associated with disinvestments in some of the less effective initiatives or those that do not fit with the priorities or agreed objectives, eg the availability of early interventions and social support for individuals who are experimenting with drugs. *Medium-term priorities* are those which require some investment to achieve clinical and structural (organizational, behavioural and management) changes, eg a comprehensive prevention programme in schools, starting at an early stage and fully involving parents. *Long-term priorities* for action may require more investment over a longer period of time, eg facilitating changes in populations' attitudes and behaviour.

Identification and pooling of resources

The key meaning of partnership in the HImP is about the ability of organizations and agencies serving a geographical area to pool their current and future resources and make them available to serve the aims and objectives of the HImP. Any future resources should be based on achievements (ie outcomes) rather than processes. Indeed, the 1998 'spending review' has linked resource allocation to achievements (ie health gain and improvements).

Accountability and responsibility

While the DAT in each locality could be the lead in developing, implementing and monitoring achievements of these HImPs, it is essential in geographical areas with more than one DAT to identify a single focal individual within the health authority to co-ordinate this. As discussed above, the substance misuse HImP will cover areas not covered by all DATs such as smoking and alcohol. This health authority individual should report to each DAT responsible for the drug action plan. However, there must be a mechanism to reconcile the statutory responsibility of the health authority enshrined under *The New NHS* legislation and the lead role of the DAT. This could be achieved by formal delegation of accountability from the health authority to the DAT. However, as there are many different agencies involved in DATs and boundaries of organizations relating to the DATs and other agencies involved in health authority HImPs are not often co-terminous, this may be difficult to achieve. The evolving roles of primary care groups (PCGs) may ensure that the monitoring of HImP-related work remains at a health authority level, perhaps addressed by public health. If this occurs, public health will have a significant role to play in co-ordinating, tracking and monitoring health-related activity within the DAT activities as well as dove-tailing substance misuse-related HImP work.

Monitoring objective implementation

There must be a clear implementation statement identifying the role of each agency, milestones, success measures and the methods by which these agencies will report to the key responsible person. Organizations, statutory or voluntary, have different management and accountability systems as well as reporting mechanisms (local authority—democratic accountability to the elected local people; health authority—central accountability to the NHS Executive; private sector—to the shareholder; voluntary sector—to the founders and management boards) and this makes monitoring a complex task.

Monitoring of health status

There will need to be clear outcome indicators to assess the overall performance of the HImP for substance misuse. Such outcome indicators could be measured in terms of[15]:

- individual outcomes (eg reduction in experimentation and use, delayed onset of use, number of patients with long remission for more than five years, etc)
- public health outcomes (eg reduction in the number of people sharing needles, HIV and hepatitis cases related to drug misuse, coronary heart disease cases, cirrhosis cases, alcohol-related admissions to A&E departments, etc)
- social outcomes (eg reduction in crime, family problems, violence associated with substance misuse) political indicators (eg increase in the number of drug seizures, positive reports on enforcement and street drug prices, reduction in number of arrests and offences related to drugs)
- health indicators (eg reduction [or increase] in referral to treatment, admission to hospital, dual diagnosis, etc).

Service provision and clinical practices

There are wide variations both in service provision for drug and alcohol misuse (Table 16.2) and clinical practices in dealing with patients (Figure 16.2). Many factors can be attributed to the variations in service provision, including lack of local strategies to deal with substance misuse, lack of clear needs assessment, changing patterns of

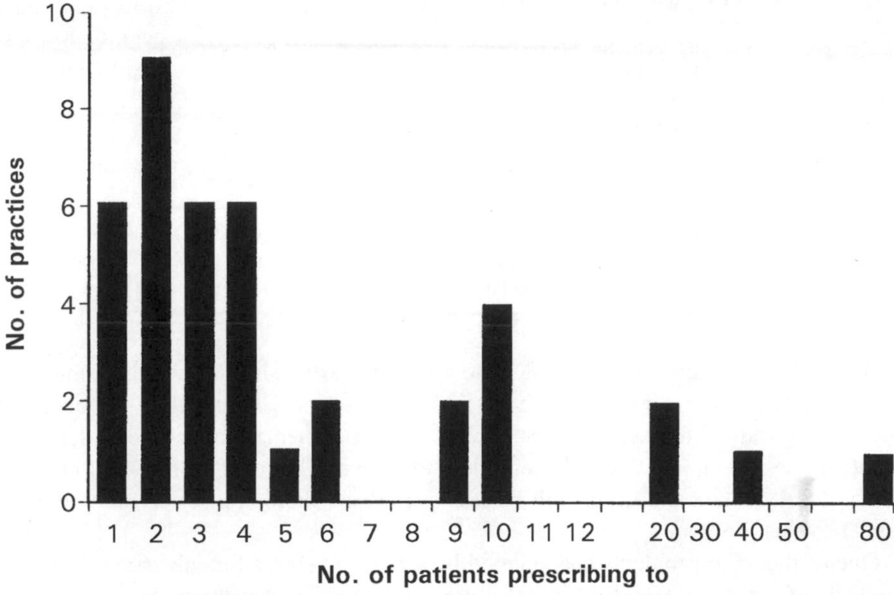

Fig. 16.2 Number of prescriptions for drug addiction according to practice in one health authority in 1998.
(Based on a survey of 136 practices in Merton, Sutton and Wandsworth Health Authority, 1998[16]).

substance use, lack of funding and scarce local expertise. Variations in clinical practice are not as easy to explain since clinical decision is based largely on a combination of scientific evidence, clinical practice and opinion (from individuals and expert groups).

Current challenges

To tackle the current scale and severity of substance misuse, decision makers and service providers must face many challenges (Table 16.3). As most traditional approaches are exhausted without any significant success, new and fresh approaches are needed. Surely the starting point is to assess and define the population's health and social needs—defining priorities and developing well resourced, comprehensive and integrated education, prevention, treatment, care and rehabilitation services to meet the identified needs.

The availability of substances and their often illicit nature is a key aspect, not shared by most other areas of healthcare. There is an increasing need for agencies such as

Table 16.2 Variation in service provision is wide

Prevention/education	is very 'patchy', and of variable quality
Treatment varies	between localities, between providers within localities, in child services, in services for women and older people

Table 16.3 Challenges to be faced

- local health and social needs assessment must be improved
- evidence of efficacy of interventions must be found
- priorities must be redefined
- services must become comprehensive and integrated
- services must become more sensitive
- a balance must be struck between the needs of individuals and
- those of the public
- national and local policies must be clarified
- professional standards must be set
- resource use should be linked to achievements

health and the criminal justice system to work in partnership. If health promotion, education and other agencies, such as the youth service, counselling services for young people and families, can assist in reducing experimentation, or at least delay the onset of use, the 'market' will become less effective. The local culture will change, demand will reduce and drugs will be less available—there is a supply and demand aspect to this problem.

One of the main problems encountered by service planners for substance misuse is the lack of appropriate and meaningful population and intervention data. This issue needs urgent attention to define the most appropriate data and its sources.

Another challenge is to balance individual and public needs. Planners and providers of services should take into account the wider impacts of drugs and alcohol on families and societies, and the aims of interventions should be the protection of the public and the elimination of harm[17].

With the multidisciplinary and agency nature of interventions in the field of substance misuse, there must be a proper system to license professionals dealing with patients and communities, with regular revalidation of these professionals and accreditation of providers, especially those dealing with young people and treatment services. This will ensure a high professional standard across the services and minimize variations in practices.

This chapter has argued that local prevalence and needs assessment studies need to be undertaken and initiatives measured according to outcomes and effectiveness. It appears that we are arguing that all initiatives should be controlled according to facts and figures. However, as we have outlined throughout, the problem is varied and complex. Qualitative approaches are also required and the different reasons why individuals and groups misuse also need teasing out, throwing light on new initiatives that may have significance for different local groups. The art as well as the science needs building into the process. This is probably the greatest challenge.

Conclusions

The HImP provides an excellent and challenging opportunity to tackle drug misuse in any given population or community. However, to develop, implement and monitor an effective HImP, organizational boundaries need to be cut across and current protective practices changed to deal with substance misuse. PCGs could and should play an important role in tackling drug misuse. Drugs can affect any individual in society directly or indirectly. Without new innovative approaches, the problem will continue to escalate as will the burden on individuals, their families and society. Finding a solution requires collaborative efforts and partnerships and HImPs provide such an opportunity. Can we capture it?

Key messages

- Use and misuse of substances (prescribed and illicit drugs, OTC drugs, alcohol and nicotine) affects individuals, their families and society as a whole; there are no age, social class, race or religion boundaries
- Substance misuse is one of the main public health and social problems facing modern societies and it has become a political priority
- Addiction is a 'chronic relapsing condition'. Prevention, therefore, is the key strategic approach to tackling the problem of drug misuse and addiction
- Since most of the traditional approaches to tackling the problems leading to increased substance use and misuse have been exhausted without any significant success, new and fresh approaches are needed
- Finding a solution requires substantial collaborative efforts and partnership and HImPs provide such an opportunity.

References

1 Ghodse AH. *Drug and addictive behaviour: a guide to treatment.* 2nd edn. Oxford: Blackwell Science, 1995.
2 Department of Health. *The task force to review services for drug misusers.* London: Department of Health, 1996.
3 Health Education Authority. *Today's young adult.* London: HEA, 1992.
4 Health Education Authority. *Tomorrow's young adult.* London: HEA, 1992.
5 Health Education Authority. *Drug realities: national drugs campaign survey.* London: HEA, 1997.
6 Department of Health. *Our healthier nation: a contract for health.* A consultative document. London: The Stationery Office, 1998. (A white paper *Saving Lives: Our Healthier Nation* was published in July 1999.)
7 Lord President. *Tackling drugs to build a better Britain.* London: The Stationery Office, 1998.
8 British Medical Association. *The Misuse of drugs.* Amsterdam: Harwood Academic, 1997.
9 Rawaf S. Public health and addiction: prevention. *Curr Opinion Psychiatry* 1998; **11**: 273–8.
10 Secretary of State for Health. *The new NHS: modern and dependable.* London: The Stationery Office, 1997.
11 Advisory Council on the Misuse of Drugs. *Treatment and rehabilitation.* London: The Stationery Office, 1984.
12 Rawaf S, Marshall F. Drug misuse; the ten steps for needs assessment. *Public Health Med* 1999; **1**: 21–6.
13 Ramsey M, Percy A. *Drug use declared Results of the 1994 British crime survey.* London: Home Office, 1996.
14 Ramsey M, Spiller J. *Drug misuse declared in 1996: Latest results from the British crime survey.* Home Office Research Study 172. London: Home Office, 1997.
15 Rawaf S, Fraser H, Oyefeso A, Ghodse H. *Predictors of treatment outcomes in drug and alcohol: a public health perspective.* Presented at the 3rd European Symposium on Drug Addiction. Istanbul, Turkey, 23–26 October 1995.
16 Rawaf S, Evans N, Floyd K. *General practitioners and drug misuse.* London: MSW Health Authority, 1998.
17 Department of Health, The Scottish Office, Welsh Office, Northern Ireland Department of Health and Social Services. *Drug misuse and dependence—Guidelines on clinical management.* London: The Stationery Office, 1999.

▶17

Minority ethnic health

Ms Veena Bahl
Department of Health Adviser on Minority Ethnic Health, UK

The Government's modernization agenda for health and social services provides an opportunity to address minority ethnic heath issues as part of the mainstream agenda of the NHS. Equity[1] and fair access are key themes and the white paper *Saving Lives: Our Healthier Nation*[2] paves the way for addressing public health issues more comprehensively through partnership approaches intended to tackle the root causes of illness and reduce inequalities in health. These include income, employment, housing, social exclusion, pollution, ethnicity and gender.

Minority ethnic groups form 7% of the UK population. The key determinants of ill health are worse for many minority ethnic communities than for the bulk of the population. As well as exhibiting marked differences compared with the Caucasian population, these groups are characterized by marked diversity in health status and disease patterns[3].

The HImP process

The white paper *The New NHS: Modern and Dependable*[4] outlines the Government's intention to build a modern and dependable health service fit for the 21st century—an NHS that works with others to improve health and reduce health inequalities. Health improvement programmes (HImPs) will be the NHS' contribution to the Government's aim of building better quality public services and strong communities. They are the local plan of action to improve health and modernize services[5].

Black and minority ethnic health has been part of the developmental agenda for a long time and there is a wealth of information available. The issue should be treated as an integral part of HImPs, which, therefore, should:

- Bring together the local NHS with local authorities and others, in particular the black and minority ethnic voluntary sector, to set a strategic framework for improving health, tackling inequalities in health which relate to ethnicity and developing more accessible, convenient, high-standard services
- Be action-focused, setting out high-level objectives and summarizing the commitments of local players, including minority ethnic community-based organizations, minority ethnic NHS staff and local authorities, to deliver these objectives
- Include measurable targets for improvement, demonstrating how resources will be used to improve the health of the population, including minority ethnic subpopulations, and modernize the NHS
- Involve all with an interest, particularly those populations such as black and minority ethnic communities who have historically had little 'voice' in the NHS.

Building black and minority ethnic health into HImPs

Black and minority ethnic health should be a key strand running through all components of HImPs.

Needs assessment

Needs assessment has been patchy and more comprehensive assessment is a key process if HImPs are to address black and minority ethnic healthcare needs. More relevant data, including data on the views of these populations, are needed to influence the development of effective HImPs.

The Department of Health is aware of the need to develop data on minority ethnic health and has taken a number of steps to address this, eg:

- census data
- contract minimum data set[6]
- epidemiological information[7]
- ethnic minorities database
- the National Institute for Ethnic Studies in Health.

Data and information held by different agencies on minority ethnic populations need to be collated. This means, for example, using the data available to the local authority on the use made of local authority services that have a significant impact on health, eg leisure facilities.

Quantitative data should be supplemented by qualitative data on the needs of minority ethnic communities, using open forums and focus groups as appropriate. Where agencies are failing to attract specific minority communities to consultative forums, they need to look at the potential of community-based organizations as a way in[8].

Resource mapping

Agencies need to share baseline information on resources and forecasts. However, the resources available to address minority ethnic issues reside in mainstream budgets, the communities and the NHS workforce, not just in project funding.

Agencies should be aware of the ethnic profile of their workforce and emerging trends, eg the decline in the proportion of nurses with minority ethnic backgrounds in the NHS, poor representation of ethnic minorities in managerial positions and growing numbers of pharmacists, opticians and doctors with a South Asian background. The local workforce needs to have the cultural competence and skills to deliver more appropriate services. Recruitment, training and development strategies must recognize the need to serve a diverse population[9]. Training needs to be multidisciplinary and involve users and carers wherever possible. The Government white paper *Working together, securing a quality workforce for the NHS* states that a key challenge is to ensure that equality of opportunity is integrated into everything the NHS does, including how staff are treated and valued[10]. Issues of racism and discrimination need to be addressed as part of the human resources strategy for the NHS.

Resources available to address minority ethnic health issues also reside in the community. Local agencies need to talk to local black and minority ethnic organizations, many of which will be well aware of the wider health and social welfare inequalities faced by their communities. They need to look at how they develop the capacity of the community to address health policy and care-delivery issues[11].

Identification of priorities for action

The NHS needs to respond to the black and minority ethnic health dimensions of the National Priorities Guidance[12]. Wherever possible, these priorities need to be translated into action that is evidence-based and intended to deliver improved outcomes.

As a *shared lead* with social services, NHS agencies need to look at the following.

Cutting health inequalities

This would include action programmes, eg to reduce the level of unwanted teenage conceptions among young African–Caribbean women and to ensure that all individuals from newly arrived communities are registered with a GP. The latter is essential if immunization targets for childhood vaccinations are to be achieved.

With respect to the development of programmes to reduce the number of accidents, plans and resources should always be developed in co-operation with people working within the communities at which those resources are targeted[12]. In providing smoking cessation services to disadvantaged groups, agencies need to be aware of differences in ethnic groups, eg the high level of smoking among Bengali populations.

Effective drug treatment and care services require awareness of social changes taking place in black and minority ethnic communities, eg as a result of cultural stereotyping, authorities may ignore emerging evidence of drug- and alcohol-related health issues among young Asian people in some parts of the country.

Mental health

There are well-known issues concerning the mental health of some minority communities, eg rate of sectioning of young African–Caribbean men, and other emerging issues, eg older Asian women presenting symptoms of depression in the GP surgery and levels of attempted suicide among younger Asian women. The most productive strategy for establishing mental health needs is to involve minority ethnic service users and carers in needs assessment[3].

Promoting independence

Rehabilitative services for people who suffer from cardiovascular disease/stroke are essential if they are to return to employment, but individuals may fall between the gaps in provision. Health agencies need to be more aware of the potential role of informal carers in some black and ethnic minority communities.

On *lead priorities* for the NHS, where social services are in support, NHS agencies need to look at the following.

Waiting lists and times

There is no national information available on waiting lists broken down by patient ethnicity. NHS agencies should consider capturing ethnic background when undertaking sampling work. This may throw up issues around local referral for specific conditions which are more prevalent in black and minority ethnic communities[1].

Primary care and dentistry

Many black and minority ethnic communities are concentrated in urban areas where primary care provision is more likely to consist of single-handed practices in poorer premises. GPs should make good use of advocacy services for minority ethnic patients given the links between good communication and effectiveness[14].

There are well-documented issues in relation to the non-uptake of dental services by minority ethnic communities[3] and reducing inequalities in access to NHS dentistry will be a significant step forward for these groups.

Coronary heart disease

It is well known that black and minority ethnic groups have a high incidence of coronary heart disease/diabetes. Women born in the Caribbean and West Africa are over 50% more likely to die of a stroke than other women.

The national service framework has set national standards and defined service models for high quality services. In the meantime, health agencies need to act on key issues for black and minority ethnic groups, including primary prevention, smoking among some of these groups and better detection. There may be real value in health visitor-led clinics to meet the needs of Asian adults at risk[3]. There is also a need for more effective rehabilitation since there are problems in integrating hospital and GP service provision.

Cancer

An appreciation of the cultural and religious issues for black and minority ethnic groups that may shape their beliefs and responses to cancer is essential in the planning and development of cancer services. It is known, for example, that the uptake of breast cancer screening services among women in some minority ethnic groups is low. Cancer primarily affects older people and overcoming language and communication barriers will be particularly important in providing effective preventive and treatment services[15].

Strategies for change

The white paper *Saving Lives: Our Healthier Nation*[2] sets out proposals for concerted action by the Government, in partnership with local organizations, to improve people's living conditions and health. In improving the health of the whole nation, a key priority will be better health for those who are worst off.

Saving Lives: Our Healthier Nation is intended to cover the spectrum of action on the wider determinants of health. For black and minority ethnic health this means working closely with local authorities which take the lead on addressing housing issues for communities more likely to live in poorer, overcrowded accommodation, lifestyle issues through appropriate provision of leisure facilities and developing integrated approaches to the development of a strong voice for black and minority ethnic community-based organizations. It means working with education services on health issues emerging among young minority ethnic people, with police services that will be more aware of emerging patterns of drug- and alcohol-related problems in some communities and with local business, including minority ethnic businesses.

In each of the four priority areas—heart disease and stroke, accidents, cancer and mental health—there are specific issues in relation to minority ethnic health that NHS agencies need to act on. The number of national targets is small and allows room for HImPs to reflect local priorities. Given that minority ethnic populations are clustered in particular areas, some authorities will, in effect, be setting minority ethnic health targets. Where there are smaller minority ethnic populations, authorities need to look at local targets that will improve health and reduce inequalities in these communities.

Healthy settings

Issues will also arise in the settings for action on health. For example, in the *healthy school setting*, effective work with black and minority ethnic pupils will need to be combined with a reduction in the disproportionate number of black pupils excluded from schools. This is an area in which combined work with local education services to reduce exclusions will be key.

Similarly, differences in employment patterns for black and minority ethnic communities present specific issues for *healthy workplace* initiatives, because members of these communities are more likely to be unemployed, self-employed, working in specific sectors of the economy and concentrated in specific parts of organizations. Awareness of these employment patterns and the ethnic profile of local workforces will be central to effectiveness in tackling health in the 'workplace'.

In *healthy neighbourhood settings*, NHS agencies need to recognize the robust networks already established in some black and minority ethnic communities and take advantage of the potential opportunities to undertake health initiatives concentrated in particular areas. In other cases, the geographical distribution of some minority ethnic communities will raise issues of how to work effectively with dispersed communities.

HImPs should include commitments to joint actions at the health and social care boundary. This will be of crucial importance to black and minority ethnic communities where community-based organizations often fill the gaps in primary, secondary, community and social service provision.

Service and financial frameworks

Service and financial frameworks for the NHS are intended to provide a robust framework for all services. Service frameworks are designed to ensure consistency, quality and accessibility. 'Quality' in healthcare for black and minority ethnic communities cannot be based solely on professional judgement—it needs to be defined with the involvement of black and minority ethnic organizations and communities.

Within these parameters, authorities need to be more rigorous in identifying and meeting local needs. It will be important that strategies are based on sound evidence of the clinical effectiveness and appropriateness of intervention. What works for one group may be inappropriate for another minority group in terms of the nature and type of mainstream services, effective clinical interventions, accessibility and appropriateness of service provision.

National framework for assessing performance

The new national framework will judge how well each part of the NHS is doing in delivering quality services. One of the key components of significance for black and minority ethnic health will be fair access to services. This will allow communities to compare performance[16]. Health agencies need to be accountable through regional offices for improving the health of black and minority ethnic communities.

Conclusions

HImPs are a vehicle for bringing about long-awaited change and improvement in the health of black and minority ethnic communities. The degree to which this is achieved is dependent on how well minority populations' expression of needs are listened to, the strength of the partnerships put in place to address these needs, and whether or not the issue becomes part of the mainstream and all available resources are used. The Government's agenda is about changing thinking and that includes changing how health and the populations served, particularly black and minority ethnic communities, are viewed.

Key messages

- Minority ethnic groups form 7% of the population
- Ethnic difference is characterized by different determinants of ill health, disease patterns, cultures, perceptions and expectations (health and illness)
- Minority ethnic health has been part of the development agenda for a long time
- In improving the health of the whole nation, a key priority will be better health for those who are worst off
- Health settings (school, work, neighbourhood, health zone) will provide greater opportunities to address minority ethnic health in collaboration with all partners for health.

References

1 Acheson D (Chairman). *Independent inquiry into inequalities in health.* London: The Stationery Office, 1998.
2 Secretary of State for Health. *Saving Lives: Our healthier nation.* London: The Stationery Office, 1999.
3 Bahl V. Ethnic minority groups. In: Rawaf S, Bahl V. *Assessing health needs of people from minority ethnic groups.* London: Royal College of Physicians, 1998; 3–19.
4 Secretary of State for Health. *The new NHS: modern and dependable.* London: The Stationery Office, 1997.
5 NHS Executive. *Health improvement programmes, planning for better health and better healthcare.* Health Service/Local Authority Circular HSC 1998/167:LAC (98) 23. Leeds: NHSE, 1998.
6 Office for Public Management. *Playing the numbers game.* London: Office for Public Management, 1996.
7 Balarajan R, Raleigh VS. *Ethnicity and health.* London: Department of Health, 1993.

8 Rawaf S, Bahl V. *Assessing health needs among people from minority ethnic groups*. London: Royal College of Physicians, 1998.
9 Chandra J. *Facing up to difference, a toolkit for creating culturally competent health services for black and minority ethnic communities*. London: King's Fund, 1996.
10 The NHS Executive. *Working together, securing a quality workforce for the NHS*. Health Service Circular HSC 1998/162.
11 Weaver M. *Developing the role of the black and minority ethnic voluntary sector in a changing NHS*. London: DOH, 1998.
12 The NHS Executive. *Modernising health and social services: national priorities guidance 1999/00–2001/02*. Leeds: NHSE, 1998.
13 Parmar A, for RoSPA. *Safety and minority ethnic communities*, 1993.
14 Yee L. *Breaking barriers towards culturally competent general practice*. London: Royal College of General Practitioners, 1997.
15 Bahl V. In: *The proceedings of the Cancer Research Campaign/Department of Health symposium on cancer and minority ethnic groups. BJC* 1996; **74**: sXXIX. London: Cancer Research Campaign, 1996.
16 Department of Health. *A first class service, quality in the new NHS*. London: DoH, 1998.

▶18

Child health

Professor Leon Polnay
Professor of Community Paediatrics, University of Nottingham, Nottingham, UK

To a community paediatrician, the shift in health policy in the direction of health improvement, enhanced quality of life and reduction in inequalities of health is initially music to the ears. In 1904, the Interdepartmental Committee on Physical Deterioration was set up by parliament to investigate the reason for the high rate of rejection of recruits to the Boer War[1]. This enlightened committee concluded that adult health was dependent on child health and made 69 recommendations on issues such as clean air, open spaces, food, exercise, juvenile smoking and alcohol use. This anticipated by nearly 100 years many of the main themes in *Health of the Nation*[2] and *Our Healthier Nation*[3]. One might cite the much older and better known example of Sodom and Gomorra when alcohol misuse, poor parenting, sexual behaviour and youth offending might also have been major concerns of the health authority of the day. The action taken and outcome might not be options available today, but they do illustrate the need to tie targets for health improvement to evidence for effective interventions.

Search for evidence-based strategies

It is relatively easy to generate a wish list of desired improvements to child health, development or wellbeing and to obtain general agreement, for example, that tobacco and alcohol use by children is harmful and should be reduced. However, 'causes' are usually multifactorial—social, economic and environmental factors are often the most important and a literature review does not yield a wealth of evidence-based effective strategies. The programme launched in optimism and enthusiasm will fail if this is not appreciated. Working with local authority partners is an essential requirement of these 'difficult to reach' targets, but this partnership is unlikely to find short-term answers to social adversity. It needs to be made clear at the outset where evidence-based solutions exist and where research and a development plan arc needed. Mrs Lot, the wife of the health authority chairman, might not have turned into a pillar of salt when, like most of us, she was tempted to watch others' misfortunes, had the Sodom and Gomorra Health Authority put its objectives into a long-term strategic plan driven by a research and development programme.

Health improvement versus illness treatment

Figure 18.1 contrasts health improvement with illness treatment. In the latter, treatment X is curative, restoring the patient to full health. Treatment Y provides only partial relief and treatment Z is ineffective. Far less is known about health

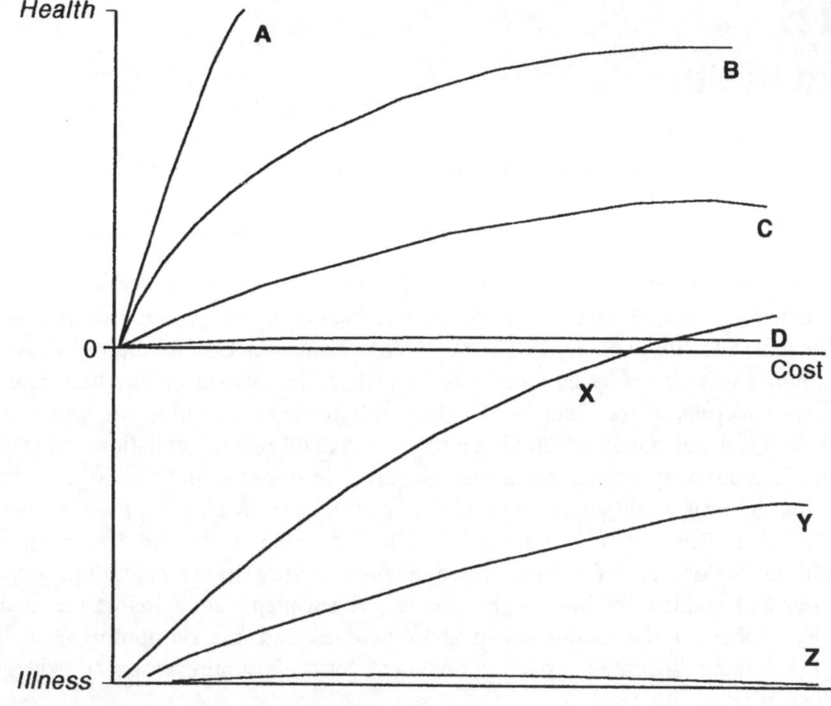

Fig. 18.1 Health improvement versus illness treatment.
The bottom half of the figure shows three different treatments X, Y and Z for treating a sick person. Treatment X is the cheapest and results in a complete cure; treatment Y is more expensive and only partly effective; treatment Z has no measurable benefit at all. The top part of the diagram uses the same sort of model applied to strategies to promote health rather than treat illness. A, B, C and D represent a range of options from A, which is cheap and effective, to D, which is expensive and produces no measurable benefit. The differences between the upper and lower parts of the figure are that we have much more evidence about what works and what doesn't work for illness treatment than we have to support decision-making in health promotion.

improvement strategies: how many (as in D) are ineffective and how many (as in A) produce impressive results in a short time and at low cost? Not many, I suspect.

'Wish list' for a health improvement programme

Figure 18.2 summarizes the pathways that should be followed from wish list through to setting realistic targets.

Child health in comparison with other branches of medicine is much better established in terms of the preventive arm of its practice with nearly a century of experience. There is a universal child health promotion programme, which over the last decade has been increasingly shaped by critical review of the available evidence[4–6]. Emphasis has shifted from screening as a major part of its content and a change of name from 'child health surveillance programme' to 'child health promotion programme'. There is a dedicated workforce to deliver it (health visitors and school nurses), although in places this has been greatly reduced on the grounds of competing health service demands.

Much of the wish list of health improvement can be found in embryo form in this programme, but for some items there is no evidence for effective interventions and for

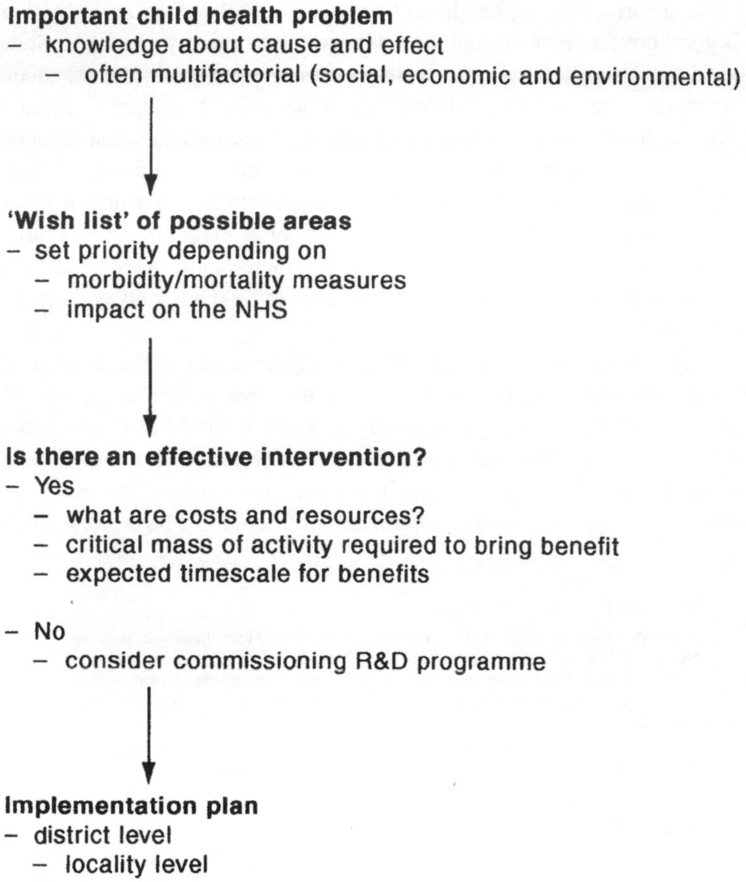

Important child health problem
- knowledge about cause and effect
  - often multifactorial (social, economic and environmental)

↓

'Wish list' of possible areas
- set priority depending on
  - morbidity/mortality measures
  - impact on the NHS

↓

Is there an effective intervention?
- Yes
  - what are costs and resources?
  - critical mass of activity required to bring benefit
  - expected timescale for benefits
- No
  - consider commissioning R&D programme

↓

Implementation plan
- district level
  - locality level

Fig. 18.2 Process for HImP.

others there may be a lack of critical mass of activity to make an impact. Health improvement is a long-term process with distant outcomes. Important long-term benefits of child health interventions may be achieved in adult physical and mental health, employment and productivity and the absence of unemployment, reliance on benefits and offending behaviours[7]. In childhood too, the lack of need for social service intervention and special education and prevention of infectious disease and accidents can greatly reduce the burden upon services. In some circumstances, prevention of a very small number of cases in which there are heavy lifelong costs might be justifiable.

Monitoring outcomes

As well as evidence of effectiveness of interventions, there is a need for a means of monitoring outcomes in the field. Reliable information to do this may not always be available. For some outcomes information is collected and reliable, eg teenage pregnancy, but might not be collated until two years or longer after the data are reported. Other information, eg height and weight, are collated on an individual basis and there is good coverage, but population data are not routinely available. Some data, eg infectious disease notifications, are available on a routine basis, but are incomplete. Other important data, eg smoking and drinking habits, are not available without special surveys. Most of the information required probably falls into this last category. The need to provide these measurement tools is a necessary precursor of the health improvement programme (HImP), together with consideration of whether or not they are needed on the whole population, a sample, yearly or at longer intervals (Table 18.1).

This information needs to be related to local characteristics, which can build up a neighbourhood profile, to enable useful comparisons to be made between one area and another (Table 18.2).

Table 18.3 records the factors that promote or impair health in the areas covered by those indicators in Table 18.1. They divide into environmental factors, lifestyle factors, parenting characteristics, parental physical and mental health, socioeconomic factors, primary and secondary prevention through an effective child health promotion programme and tertiary prevention through effective treatment of illness. Table 18.4 lists priority areas for child health improvement plans[8]. These were derived in

Table 18.1 Desert island data

A suggested short, but useful and informative, dataset, derived from the principles of the BBC *Desert Island Disks* radio programme in which distinguished people are asked to select just eight pieces of music which they would choose to have with them if marooned on a desert island. The current list partly derives from the selections of a group of community paediatricians given a similar task.

Accidents	Asthma admissions
Notified infections	Alcohol
Height/weight	Smoking
Diets	Substance misuse
Self-harm	Exercise
Sexually transmitted diseases	Youth offences
Teenage pregnancy	School absence: illness, truancy
Child protection	Special educational needs

Table 18.2 Local characteristics

Environment
Population
Employment
Income
Neighbourhood characteristics*
Family structures
Service provision
Service access

*eg: age, quality, type and tenure of housing; urban, rural; working class, middle class; proportion of single, elderly; new community, stable community, high mobility; community identity, events organisations, level of inclusion/exclusion; dominant cultures; deprivation indices; etc

Sydney, Australia using strict criteria to rank the importance of candidate areas. The lower part of the table lists those evidence-based interventions that could be applied to those target areas.

Implementation of a HImP for children

Size of the task

How can a HImP for children be implemented? Many of the target areas in the shopping basket will vary greatly from one general practice to another, from locality to locality and from school to school (see Tables 18.3 and 18.4). They will be strongly related to social adversity. Some might be improving within a neighbourhood without any intervention; in others some might be worsening. The size of the task facing different areas may vary greatly (Figure 18.3). Area A already exceeds the target—areas B and C do not. Viewed at a district level, area C may contribute a large component of the total burden of morbidity in a particular category. Information must therefore be available at a local level (school, practice, neighbourhood, primary care group, ward) and be delivered on a regular and timely basis to those working in the HImP. This might take the form of a profile involving a number of health indicators. Without this, local and individual problems and achievements are invisible. Informed discussion at a local level with the establishment of local alliances is needed to determine the relative priorities for different areas in the district strategy. Locality profiles will greatly assist in establishing local needs and planning programmes most appropriately for that particular area.

Table 18.3 Factors that can be expected to have a positive or negative influence on child health in a locality

Impair	Promote
Environment	*HImP*
Food	Immunization
Water	Screening tests
Air	Health promotion and accident prevention advice
Noise	*Cure of illness versus complications, residual disability*
Temperature	Prompt treatment
Dampness	Effective treatment
Overcrowding	*Effects of poverty*
Home safety	Maternal ill health and depression
Road safety	*Parenting characteristics*
School safety	Protection
Recreation safety	Care
Lifestyle	Security
Exercise	Stimulation
Smoking	Love
Alcohol	Support
Substance misuse	Education and training
Sexually transmitted diseases	Example
	Commitment
	Consistency

Table 18.4 Important areas in child health which a HImP might target. These were the highest priority areas identified by Sydney Areas Health Service[8] and are very similar to current targets in recent UK policy

- Tobacco
- Alcohol and drugs
- Low birth weight and prematurity
- Perinatal and infant mortality
- Self-harm
- Depression
- Conduct disorder
- Sexuality
- Child abuse
- Attention deficit hyperactivity disorder
- Sunlight
- Infection—immunization
- Domestic violence
- Learning difficulties
- Nutrition
- Social/environment
- Parents with mental illness

Evidence-based interventions

- Home visiting programmes
- Health promoting schools
- Early intervention programmes
- Multidisciplinary assessment and therapy, eg in learning difficulties
- Public education programmes
- Community-based programmes
- Health worker education and continuing medical education
- Advocacy and lobbying
- Targeted screening

Local leadership

Leadership and commitment need to be provided and sustained at a local level over the long term. This is easy to achieve in area A (Figure 18.3), but is progressively more difficult in areas B and C where the challenges for healthcare professionals will be much greater and the effort and resources required to bring about change considerably higher. A familiar example would be the effort needed to obtain a high level of immunization in a deprived area compared to an affluent area. Morale can easily suffer under the burden of a seemingly impossible task. There is a need to recognize when resources are not up to the task. It is essential to have external support, staff training, feedback of results and a carefully designed programme that is feasible within the resources, skills and time-scale applied. Areas A, B and C are not equal in their needs, but too often resources are allocated related to population size rather than need.

Solid collaboration

Programmes can flounder, especially where they involve multiple agencies and there is difficulty in finding agreement over how the costs of the programme might be

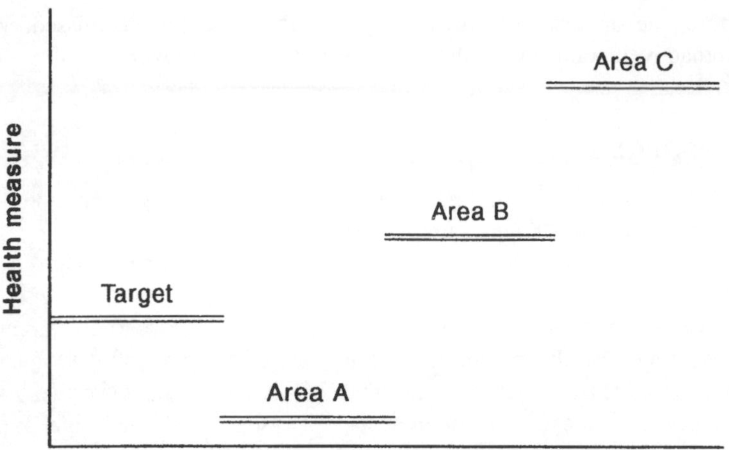

Fig. 18.3 Variation in locality health promotion needs.

shared, eg between education services and health. This is a major difficulty at a time when all services are looking for savings rather than expenditure and competing demands are made for their time, eg literacy hour for schools. Continuity of policy and practice over longer periods of time may be difficult to sustain in the face of changing political, professional and financial pressures. High staff turnovers, which often occur in the areas of greatest need and pressure, can also impede continuity of practice, programme and collaboration.

Long-term perspective

In the long term, success is achieved through individual optimism, courage, enthusiasm and commitment. Local practitioners need to be creative in modifying policies and their implementation to meet local population needs. It should be appreciated that the HImP for children requires a long-term perspective, a commitment to inter-agency working and an understanding that the most important outcomes may take years to be seen, eg in adult life or even the next generation.

Conclusions

The health of the future generation should be the cornerstone of any HImP aiming at long-term investment in the public's health. While causes of ill health are multifactorial, the social, economic and environmental elements are often the most important. Important health problems and their antecedents can be recognized; for some there is evidence for effective interventions, for others research is needed. New information systems may need to be set up to ensure that baseline and outcome measures are recorded.

Solid partnership to achieve change and consolidate improvement is essential. Such partnership should be consolidated through a visionary leadership and sustained commitment at local level over the long term. Priorities for child health are known and, therefore, the opportunity provided by HImP should not be missed. What is needed is proactive action (rather than reaction) at the local level.

Key messages

- Causes of ill health are multifactorial: social, economic and cnvironmental factors, yet effective strategies are scarce
- Preventive child health, in comparison with other areas of medicine, is well established
- While the effectiveness of treatment can be predicted, less is known about the effectiveness of HImP strategies: how many are ineffective and how many are producing impressive results? As well as evidence of effectiveness on interventions, a means of monitoring outcomes is needed, but reliable information may not always be available
- Social adversity is a key determinant of what needs targeting in each GP practice
- The health improvement of children requires a long-term perspective, a commitment to interagency working and an appreciation that the most important outcomes may be many years hence in adult life or even in the next generation.

References

1 Interdepartmental Committee on Physical Deterioration. *Parliamentary report*, vol 1 [cd 2175], vol 2 [cd 2210], vol 3 [cd 21860]. London: The Stationery Office, 1904.
2 Department of Health. *The health of the nation: a strategy for health in England.* London: The Stationery Office, 1992.
3 Department of Health. *Our healthier nation: a contract for health.* A consultative document. London: The Stationery Office, 1998.
4 Hall DMB, ed. *Health for all children.* 1st ed. Oxford: Oxford University Press, 1989.
5 Hall DMB, ed. *Health for all children.* 2nd ed. Oxford: Oxford University Press, 1991.
6 Hall DMB, ed. *Health for all children.* 3rd ed. Oxford: Oxford University Press, 1996.
7 Schweindart LJ, Weihart DP. *Young children grown up. The effects of the Perry pre-school programme on youth through age 15.* Ypsilanti MI, ed. Monographs of High Scope Educational Research Programme no 7. High Scope Education & Research Foundation, 1980.
8 Alperstein G, Nossar V. Key interventions for the health improvement of children and youth: a population-based approach. *Ambulatory Child Health* 1998;**4**: 295–306.
9 Polnay L (Chairman). *Health needs of school age children.* A report of a working group. London: British Paediatric Association, 1995: 28–30.

▶19

Older people's health

Professor Anthea Tinker

Professor of Social Gerontology, King's College London, and President, Section of Geriatrics and Gerontology, Royal Society of Medicine, London, UK

Health improvement programmes (HImPs) are 'local strategies for improving health and healthcare and delivering better integrated care' where it is intended that health authorities should be in the lead but 'work in partnerships with a wide range of local interests'[(1)]. As far as older people are concerned, three questions need to be asked before the issues of policies, organization and involvement are discussed.

Three questions to set the scene

1. Why should older people be singled out for separate discussion?

There are a number of cogent reasons for specifically considering older people:

- *Demographic pressures* of an ageing population (ie proportionately more older people in the population and more very old)[(2)]. However, these increases must not be exaggerated
- *Particular medical problems* are more prevalent in the older age group: there is clear evidence of a greater incidence of both acute and chronic sickness among older people compared with other age groups[(3)]. There are also differences in the way older people react to disease (eg pain mechanisms). General background, too, has an effect, eg poverty, lack of status and disability can all lead to depression, which is a major but underestimated problem. Although generalizations are dangerous, there are some special needs that must be considered, including older women, people from minority ethnic groups and homeless older people. These are all issues for which GPs and social service departments need to co-ordinate their actions
- The growing power of this group reflected in its potential *voting power*. A new generation is also becoming more articulate and learning from the Disability Lobby[(3)]
- *Rising expectations*
- *Previous neglect of this group*.

2. What can be learned from past initiatives?

When considering any initiative, it is salutary to put it in context by looking at the past. A change of language does not necessarily mean a change of policy, eg from 'a seamless service' to 'joined-up government'.

The circular advising on HImPs states that 'they do not begin from a blank sheet'[(4)]—there have been many attempts to provide co-ordinated policies and services, eg joint consultative committees[3]. To overcome some of the problems when health, social and other budgets are separate, which increases the likelihood of cost shunting, lessons can be learned from *joint finance*; this is the special allocation of money to health authorities which they can allocate to local authorities and other organizations for specific joint-care programmes[1]. However, this money has increasingly been used to pump prime new services with social services departments picking up the tab in the long run. There is now a need to see partnerships between services as joint working and not a peripheral activity.

Numerous innovations and initiatives have often not lasted beyond the short lifetime of the project nor been evaluated. However, useful lessons have come from the *Health of the Nation* initiative[5]. An evaluation welcomed this as the first attempt to put in place a national strategy based on the WHO initiative *Health for All*[6]. However, it has failed to reach its full potential and, while its impact on policy documents peaked in 1993, at local level it was negligible. It was found that shared ownership of the strategy was missing both nationally and locally. There was no major readjustment in investment priorities but health promotion did increase over five years and then tailed off. It had no serious impact on primary care practitioners and problems arose from the different cultures and agendas of health and local authorities.

3. How will these programmes link up with future initiatives on older people?

A number of initiatives are or will be relevant, eg 1999 is the United Nations' Year of Older People and the year the Royal Commission on Long Term Care of Elderly People will report. The increased emphasis on the participation of older people in policies and research is also likely to be a key influence.

Applying HImPs to older people

Attention has now turned to HImPs and older people under three broad headings:

- What should the policies be?
- How are these programmes to be organized?
- Who should be involved?

1. What should the policies be?

The objectives of HImPs have to be seen in the context of *The New NHS*[2] and *Saving Lives: Our Healthier Nation*[7] and are to:

- improve health
- tackle inequalities (with an acceptance that these are wider than in *Saving Lives: Our Healthier Nation*[7])
- develop faster, more convenient services of a consistently high standard (but what does this mean and how can it be measured?).

In *Saving Lives: Our Healthier Nation*, four priorities are set out:

- heart disease and stroke
- accidents

- cancer
- mental health.

The first and third of these targets are specifically for those aged 65 and under. Why are older people not included? Also, could not the overall targets be more specific, eg fractured neck of femur or reducing the incidence of accidents from osteoporosis? In West Essex, 'depression in older people' is a mental health category, indicating that older people are not neglected by everybody.

But the two key aims are very important for older people, ie:

- to improve the health of the population as a whole by increasing the length of people's lives and the number of years people spend free from illness
- to improve the health of the worst off in society and to narrow the health gap.

It is also good that of the three settings described one is a healthier neighbourhood with an emphasis on older people. The others are schools and workplaces. Also to be welcomed are the proposed appointment of a Minister of Public Health and health impact statements(7).

The key health services for older people are:

- *primary*—a good and sensitive service which includes prevention
- *acute care*
- *assessment and reassessment*
- *prevention*—the Social Services white paper(8) proposes giving local authorities a:
  - *partnership grant* which includes emphasis on rehabilitation 'avoiding unnecessary admissions to hospital and other institutional care, improving discharge arrangements'
  - *prevention grant* to promote independence 'so as to target some low level support for people most at risk of losing their independence' and 'encouraging an approach which helps people do things for as long as possible in their own home'.

However, at all levels one of the most important points is to counter the clear evidence of age discrimination in health services(9,10).

How are these programmes to be organized?

In developing an integrated and effective HImP specific to the needs of older people, a number of issues must be considered.

The impact of national policies on older people

The growing unacceptability of local inequalities, such as the number of hip replacements, is leading to national priorities but these have to be balanced by 'locally determined needs'(4). Some national initiatives which will have a local impact include the *Interministerial Group*. In its 1998 consultation paper *Building a Better Britain for Older People*, three areas are identified as priorities for work across government: promoting active ageing, improving care and ensuring that the Government listens to, consults and involves older people in the development of policy and the delivery of services(11). The *Better Government for Older People* initiative is a central programme under the Cabinet Office, which will run for two years and will be followed by a *Best*

Practice Guide. It will develop and test integrated strategies on the ground and examine innovative ways of delivering services in a co-ordinated and user-friendly way. In all, 28 pilot projects have been set up around the country covering all the public services that older people deal with regularly. The aims are to:

- simplify access to services
- improvc thc links between services
- provide clearer and more accessible information on older people's rights
- give older people more input into the types of services they can get and make better use of their contributions.

The ideal role, size and structure for the provision of local health and other services

In the Department of the Environment, Transport and the Regions white paper *Modernising Local Government: In touch with the people* there is recognition 'that local authorities have a key role to play as the leaders of their communities'[(12)]. As for health, the HImPs advisory circular 167/98 states that it will involve local authorities more and it will also offer them 'greater insight and a stronger voice in the formative stages of NHS service plans'[(4)].

Regarding size and structure, will there be a more fundamental change in the structure of health and local services such as regional government? With devolution in Scotland and Wales this must, at least, be an option. But how acceptable would an elected body be to those involved in health? In the immediate future there is the issue of overlap of boundaries between HImPs and local authorities which could pose problems.

Bringing it all together—the importance of a co-ordinated approach

To achieve the aims of HImPs (ie needs assessment, resource mapping, identification of priorities for action, strategies for change and a service and financial framework for the NHS), there will have to be a co-ordinated approach. One way is through pooled budgets[(1)].

Structures are important but people are more important

There is a need to match HImPs with greater understanding between professionals by joint training, multidisciplinary conferences, secondments, etc.

Who should be involved?

The objectives of HImPs give guidance on who should be involved: 'to bring together the local NHS with local authorities and others, including the voluntary sector, to set the strategic framework (for improving health, tackling inequalities and developing faster, more convenient services of a consistently high standard)'[(4)] and to 'lead local alliances'[(13)]. The local NHS must include primary care groups (PCGs) and health action zones. The groups to be brought in are older people themselves, carers, local authorities and other relevant services and professionals.

Bringing in older people

In the development of social policy, older people are reasonably represented among members of parliament and local councillors. In the health service, older people may represent their own views or an organization may do this on their behalf. If the former, then how individuals are chosen is an issue, eg PCGs have advertised for lay members. The method seems to be self-identification followed by interview by the health authority. It is unclear how such a process can identify people who have been authorized and empowered by users and carers to speak on their behalf.

There is a difference between consultation and involvement[(14)]. In this context the guidance for local authorities on methods of involving the public is helpful[(15)]:

- seeking the views of the citizen, eg juries, focus groups, conferences, opinion poll (where councils introduce lay experience and views to their decision making)
- recognizing communities by increasing their involvement in direct decision making, eg forums or managing housing services
- enabling the electorate to determine or influence policy on a specific issue, eg referendum
- watchdog or scrutiny role for the citizen, eg the right to ask for papers
- opening up the authority, eg public question time/inviting members of the public on to committees.

Working with carers

Carers are increasingly being involved. The largest group of co-resident carers is spouses who are usually also old. A consultation/white paper is expected in 1999 on a National Carers Strategy.

Role of local authorities

There is rethinking on the role of local authorities which includes that of 'promoting the economic, social and environmental wellbeing of their areas'[(16)]. This fits in with the guidance on HImPs which states 'this will engage the local authority corporately, since action on the determinants of health will span the range of local authority responsibilities: for example, housing, transport, education, environment, leisure'[(4)].

In local authorities the role of social services is also likely to change following the 1998 white paper *Modernising Social Services*[(8)]. One of most important links must be for HImP programmes to work with social services plans for community care.

Bringing in other relevant services and professionals

An objective of HImPs is to 'work with partner organizations and professionals'[(4)]. A wide range of agencies must be included. The role of *housing* for older people is vital and this includes mainstream as well as specialist housing. The Department of Health/Department of the Environment *Housing and Community Care: Establishing a Strategic Framework*[(17)] and a workbook[(18)] gives guidance for practitioners in housing, health and social services with examples of what each needs to understand and can expect of the other. It is also important to include services concerned with income, transport and mobility. The independent sector (private and voluntary) should also be included. Other, less obvious, professionals who should be involved include sheltered housing wardens.

Conclusions

Many of the features of HImPs are welcome to older people.

- *Quality and standards*: this is also the main emphasis in *A First Class Service: Quality in the New NHS*[19]. The latter includes fair access on the grounds of age, ethnicity, sex and patient/carer's experience. On standards this fits in with the Department of Education, Transport and the Regions' advice[15,16] and with the Social Services white paper[8]. The latter includes measures of the *effectiveness* of service delivery and outcomes (eg the number of households receiving intensive home care per 1000 households with members over the age of 75), *cost efficiency* (eg unit costs), *national priorities and strategic objectives* (eg emergency admissions to hospital of people aged 75 and over, and fair access, such as people aged 65 and over enabled to live at home)
- *Co-ordination*
- *Commitment to the involvement of patients and carers.*

What must also be addressed, however, is the inequalities in services and rationing of health resources accompanying the move towards capped budgets. By looking at key areas where progress could be made and where there is good practice, such as hospital discharge, HImPs could prove a useful vehicle for change.

Key messages

- Demographic changes, political power and higher expectations of older people will influence many of the actions on the future health agenda
- Health authorities, PCGs and NHS trusts should listen to and involve older people in policy formulation, decision making and service delivery and not rely solely on the formality of consultations
- HImPs for older people should balance local and national policies
- Pooled budgets could be one approach to co-ordinating services between health and local government
- Using current good practices, HImPs could prove a useful vehicle for change.

References

1 Department of Health. *Partnerships in action: new opportunities for joint working between health and social services.* A discussion document. London: DoH, 1998.
2 Secretary of State for Health. *The new NHS: modern and dependable.* London: The Stationery Office, 1997.
3 Tinker A. *Older people in modern society.* 4th ed. London: Addison, Wesley Longman, 1997.
4 Department of Health. *Health improvement programmes: planning for better health and better healthcare.* HSC 1998/167: LAC (98) 23. London: DoH, 1998.
5 Department of Health. *The health of the nation: a strategy for health in England.* London: The Stationery Office, 1992.

6 Universities of Leeds and Glamorgan and London School of Hygiene and Tropical Medicine. *The health of the nation—A policy assessed*. London: The Stationery Office, 1998.
7 Secretary of State for Health. *Saving lives: our healthier nation*. London: The Stationery Office, 1999.
8 Department of Health. *Modernising social services: promoting independence, improving protection, raising standards*. London: The Stationery Office, 1998.
9 McEwen E. Age: *the unrecognised discrimination*. London: Age Concern England, 1990.
10 Grimley Evans J. The menace of ageism: a call to arms. AC Comfort memorial lecture. Royal Society of Medicine, 15th March 1997.
11 Department of Social Security. *Building a better Britain for older people*. London: DSS, 1998.
12 Department of the Environment, Transport and the Regions. *Modernising local government: in touch with the people*. London: The Stationery Office, 1998.
13 Department of Health. *Target: our healthier nation. Faith, health and communities*. Issue 31. London: DoH, 1998.
14 Fereday G. Health improvement programme and the public. In: Rawaf S, Orton P, eds. *Health improvement programmes: the millennium approach to health and healthcare*. London: Royal Society of Medicine, 1999: ch 8.
15 Department of the Environment, Transport and the Regions. *Modernising local government: local democracy and community leadership*. London: DETR, 1998.
16 Department of the Environment, Transport and the Regions. *Modernising local government: improving local services through best value*. London: DETR, 1998.
17 Department of Health and Department of the Environment, Transport and the Regions. *Housing and community care: establishing a strategic framework*. London: DoH/DETR, 1997.
18 Means R, Brenton M, Harrison L, Heywood F. *Making partnerships work in community care: a guide for practitioners in housing, health and social services*. London: DoH/DETR, 1997.
19 Department of Health. *A first class service: quality in the new NHS*. London: DoH, 1998.

▶ 20

The current approach: strengths, weaknesses and the way forward

Mr Gerald Jones
Chief Executive, Wandsworth Borough Council, London, UK

Dr Salman Rawaf
Director of Clinical Standards/Senior Lecturer, Merton, Sutton and Wandsworth Health Authority, London, UK

Many health reforms and improvements have been jettisoned because they did not deliver visible results at a speed in line with political expectations. Others were merely lost due to the overlaying of a welter of further policy initiatives, each making additional demands on the requirements of policy makers, managers and medical staff. Improving healthcare, however, requires a long-term commitment and HImPs must be given time to develop and prove themselves if they are not to follow the path of some earlier initiatives into ultimate obscurity.

This final chapter attempts an overview of the health improvement programme (HImP) approach, looking particularly at its strengths and weaknesses in the current climate of British health policy. It identifies factors that are likely to be critically important in the success of HImPs—investment levels and resources, cultural changes and partnership working, achievement of long-term commitments at local level and awareness of the role of individual citizens in health improvement.

The strengths and weaknesses identified for discussion are merely the most important ones. Strengths are considered to be:

- sound and reasonable aims
- proper structure
- linkage of key partners—health and local authority, community
- consultation built in
- three-year development time-scale indicated.

Weaknesses or threats are considered to be:

- competing initiatives and reforms
- resources and investment
- difficulties of tackling some types of inequality
- difficulties of partnership working.

Strengths

Sound and reasonable aims

Generally, the aims of the HImP process are well thought out and comprehensive[(1)]. The link to the *Our Healthier Nation* targets provides sound continuity with earlier and parallel policy[2,3]. The emphasis on producing a strategic framework is highly desirable. HImPs are ambitious perhaps in aiming towards 'tackling inequalities and developing faster, more convenient services of a consistently high target'[1,4,5]. The potential problems of inequalities and resources/investment are highlighted below.

Proper structure

HImPs have been given the proper structure of a classic planning cycle—stating needs and objectives, identifying improvements that are required and settling the resources, targets and actions (by various parties) needed for achievement. Subsequently, monitoring and rolling forward the plan takes place. Full local consultation is required with all local agencies and populations. While this gives the various contributors and practitioners a very full workload and a requirement for extensive documentation, it is essential that most, if not all, of the planning phases are properly included, especially the monitoring phase. This latter phase, if followed through, will allow non-achievement and poor performance areas to be identified as in need of action rather than HImPs being left to gather dust on the shelves.

Linkage of key partners

HImPs build on the growing trend for whole community health improvement and follow earlier and current efforts, such as healthy alliances and health-promoting primary schools. These recognized the major contributions that local authorities could make to health improvements via their leisure, housing, environmental regulatory and publicity programmes, as well as the key role of schools and colleges in putting health education issues firmly onto the curriculum. The voluntary sector and community organizations also have a key role to play if health improvement is successfully to tackle 'lifestyle' issues. Other agencies such as the police and probation service have significant contributions to make to areas such as drug and alcohol misuse and accidents.

Built-in consultation

This is a particularly essential part of the planning process given the rather limited membership of health authority and trust boards—and their lack of local democratic involvement.

Three-year development time-scale

Given the extensive scope of HImPs and their essentially long-term objectives it is essential to allow a fairly significant period of development. A three-year period gives some measure of certainty and should help achieve the necessary commitment from all agencies. However, full development and demonstrable results are likely to take considerably longer.

Weaknesses and threats

Competing initiatives and reforms

As well as developing HImPs, the NHS is simultaneously seeking to develop primary care groups (PCGs) and trusts, abolish the internal market including fundholding, establish clinical governance principles and work towards national standards. Furthermore, it is charged to introduce specific projects, such as NHS Direct, and continue with the private finance initiative for all major capital projects, as well as many other initiatives. All these demand immense time and energy from key managers and lead professionals. There are also real issues of management and practitioner time and resources for key partners who have their own equally demanding agenda of change—local government, for example, has its 'modernizing' agenda, crime audits, youth offending teams, 'best value' and liaison with the new regional development agencies. With these competing pressures there is a danger of HImPs being marginalized and starved of effort and resources.

Resources and investment

HImPs are being introduced at a time when there is tremendous pressure on resources for healthcare. Three key factors have been identified as contributing to a medical inflation of some 10% in real terms:

- New technology is generating need (defined as where benefits can reasonably be expected from intervention) and increased professional and patient expectations. Both biological and therapeutic technologies are growing at an incredible rate and in all directions. These will widen the base for those who will benefit from the intervention and thus need and demand it. Examples such as treatment for traumatic disorders, dementia, genetic disorders and in oncology are legion. There is also an expectation of enhanced treatment for illnesses and diseases for which currently there are limited treatments (eg mental disorders, multiple sclerosis and many cancers)
- Life expectancy is increasing rapidly, causing a greater percentage of the population to occupy the age bands which make high or very high demands on NHS resources. Since 1970, the life expectancy of 60-year-olds has risen from 78 to 84 years in men and from 82 to 88 years in women
- Other NHS-dependent population groups, particularly those with multiple disability or other highly demanding conditions, are showing greatly improved survival rates, again pressurizing resources.

Problems of tackling some types of inequality

HImPs rightly prioritize the reduction of health inequalities, reflecting the earlier proposal to do so in *Saving Lives: Our Healthier Nation*[(2,3)]. However, inequalities arise from various sources that need to be differentiated. They can be due to variations in:

- the NHS, on standards, local policy, existing services (acute and primary care)
- the NHS, in matching new resources to needs
- health risks in the local environment due to pollution, etc
- access to health-related opportunities—housing, employment, education
- other health-related factors—income, social factors, etc.

Research has shown that the level of education attained is one of the major correlates with an individual's health[(6,7)]. Many of the inequalities of opportunity such as income

Role of the individual citizen in creating a healthier environment

Most environmental, social and economic factors which lead to ill health and social disharmony (including exclusion) are manmade. The role of individuals in improving the population's health is therefore extremely important. Preparing children for citizenship and promoting their understanding of the factors contributing to a healthy lifestyle and environment are essential if in the future they are to endeavour to protect the environment, to have a healthy social network and support and, above all, to protect and promote their own health.

Major attempts are already being made to include the more obvious elements of health awareness into the education process at primary school level: drugs, smoking, alcohol, teenage pregnancy, good diet and the importance of exercise are all standard features of the health education curriculum. Agenda 21 and environmental and pollution issues are also well covered in junior schools, as, increasingly, are citizenship issues themselves and topics such as crime prevention and antisocial behaviour.

Is there hope of improvement for the individual from such education programmes? The answer must be carefully qualified at this stage. Taking drug misuse as an example, what constitutes an effective drug education programme has yet to be demonstrated: longitudinal studies—which take time and are expensive—will be needed to pinpoint the best approaches. Some commentators remain cynical that great benefits will derive from this source, given cultural and peer group pressures on today's youth to sample drugs as well as the financial rewards for illegal supply. However, the consensus must remain that education programmes aimed at the individual are essential and research to develop the most effective delivery methods must be driven forward and analysed.

Long-term commitment at the local level

This is a different principle entirely, picking up on the simultaneous benefits and challenges of partnership working. To ensure that HImPs deliver health gain it is vital that the consultation benefits and contributions from partners are picked up. This requires that the difficulties of partnership working are faced and a long-term commitment made to overcome them and to achieve results. The monitoring process will be vital to demonstrate that all agencies are participating and delivering their contributions. Given the cultural differences and other problems identified above, this process is going to take time and success will therefore demand a long-term commitment from leaders, chairmen and top management of all agencies.

Conclusions

We remain optimistic about the very great potential of HImPs. This book illustrates the very great range of issues and challenges involved and this paper distils out the key strengths, weaknesses and important principles. Central to success are long-term commitment, continued investment and a careful balance between treatment and prevention and perseverance to obtain the maximum benefits from all agencies in the difficult arena of partnership working.

Key messages

- HImPs will fail unless they deliver visible results at a speed in line with political expectations
- The HImP process is well thought out and comprehensive
- Addressing inequalities and resource/investment are potential problems
- Successful HImPs should build on the growing trend for whole community health improvement and follow earlier and current efforts, eg healthy alliances
- Given the extensive scope of HImPs and their essentially long-term objectives, it is essential to allow a fairly significant period of development
- Long-term commitments, therefore, should guide health policies and investments.

References

1 Secretary of State for Health. *The new NHS: modern and dependable.* London: The Stationery Office, 1997.

2 Secretary of State for Health. *Our healthier nation: a contract for health.* A consultative paper. London: The Stationery Office, 1998.

3 Secretary of State for Health. *Saving lives: our healthier nation.* London: The Stationery Office, 1999.

4 Acheson D (Chairman). *Independent inquiry into inequalities in health.* London: The Stationery Office, 1998.

5 Department of Health. *Reducing health inequalities: an action report.* London: Department of Health, 1999.

6 Bynner J, Parsons S. *It doesn't get any better: the impact of poor basic skills on the lives of 37 year olds.* London: The Basic Skills Agency, 1997.

7 Montgomery S, Schoon I. Health and health behaviour. In: Bynner J, Ferri E, Shepherd P, eds. *Twenty something in the 1990s: getting on, getting by, getting nowhere.* Aldershot: Ashgate, 1997.

8 Marmot M, Ryff C, Bumpass L *et al.* Social inequalities in health: next questions and converging evidence. *Soc Sci Med* 1997; **44**: 901–10.

▶ Appendix 1

Clinical governance: the system and its components (tools)

Dr Salman Rawaf

Director of Clinical Standards/Senior Lecturer, Merton, Sutton and Wandsworth Health Authority, London, UK

Dr Kelly Powell

Specialist Registrar in Public Health Medicine, Merton, Sutton and Wandsworth Health Authority, London, UK

Individuals and communities who are interested in maintaining a healthy lifestyle and politicians who decide on the use of national and local resources expect that clinicians are competent and up to date in their practice. They should be supported by strong organizations which aim to improve health and meet need.

The white paper *The New NHS: Modern and Dependable*[1] stated the Government's concern with inconsistent, poor quality clinical care and for the first time gave all health organizations in the NHS a statutory duty to seek quality improvement through a defined system of 'clinical governance'.

While using the main components (tools) of the clinical governance system is relatively straightforward in NHS trusts, it is less so for primary care groups (PCGs) and public health practitioners.

Definition

Clinical governance is 'a system through which all of the organizations in the NHS are accountable for continuously improving the quality of their clinical services and ensuring high standards of patient care by creating a facilitative environment in which excellence will flourish'[2]. It:

- is basically a framework for the improvement of patient care through commitment to high standards, reflective practice, risk management and personal and team development
- is about providing the best possible clinical care for patients, identifying and avoiding areas of high risk in patient care and making the most effective use of available resources
- is about the balance between individual clinical responsibility and the collective responsibility of the team, service or organization
- for the first time, places a statutory duty for quality of care on healthcare managers equal to their pre-existing duty of financial responsibility.

To develop a NHS in which there is fair access to consistently high-quality healthcare for all, the following components have been identified as necessary[1,2]:

- clear national standards
- mechanisms for ensuring local delivery of these standards
- mechanisms for monitoring the delivery of these standards.

Standards will be set at a national level with the development of National Service Frameworks (NSFs) and the National Institute for Clinical Excellence (NICE). It will, obviously, take time to cover all of the important areas of healthcare, so, in many clinical areas, local standards will be set in the intervening period. These local standards must be shown to be based on the best available evidence.

Mechanisms to ensure local delivery of these clinical standards are the responsibility of the local trusts and the health authority (for PCGs). However, it must be recognized that changing the clinical behaviour of individual practitioners will require a variety of interventions. A complex process has to be planned at the early stages of medical education and should include altering the structure in which clinicians train and work.

Monitoring of these standards will be undertaken both locally (by trusts, the health authority and PCGs) and nationally (by the Commission for Health Improvement and the National Survey of Patient and User Experiences).

Rationale

The white paper *The New NHS: Modern and Dependable*[(1)] stated the Government's concern with inconsistent, poor quality clinical care. The 1990 NHS reforms put the emphasis on finance and stimulated quantity- rather than quality-driven competition. This was highlighted by a number of well-publicized serious failures in clinical care, such as the Bristol paediatric cardiothoracic deaths and failures in breast and cervical cancer screening, and made worse by obviousl, but hard-to-explain, variations in standards and clinical care and by major inquiries into service failures. To regain public confidence and trust, it was necessary to emphasize the importance of clinical quality, hence the inception of clinical governance. However, it is important to realize that clinical governance does not imply entirely new activity but can incorporate existing systems.

Necessary tools

There are a number of tools (components) that can be used in the three areas of setting (identifying), applying and monitoring standards (Table A1.1). To operate an effective and smooth-running clinical governance system, these components must be interlinked and work interdependently (Figure A1.1 and Table A1.2). The role of management is to ensure system maintenance ('oiling the system'), clear lines of accountability, transparency of reporting and action to implement change. The main tools are described below.

Clinical audit

This is a very important tool for clinical governance, but it is important that audit does not become the goal itself. Instead, it should be used to encourage clinicians to work to preset standards, and frequently review the quality of care they provide, making

Table A1.1 Tools available to set (identify), apply and monitor standards

Identify standards	Apply standards	Monitor standards
Evidence-based medicine	Manpower planning	Clinical audit
Clinical standards	Continuing professional development and lifelong learning	National inquiries
Research and development	Job plan	Complaints
	Risk management	Monitoring and evaluation
		Whistle-blowing

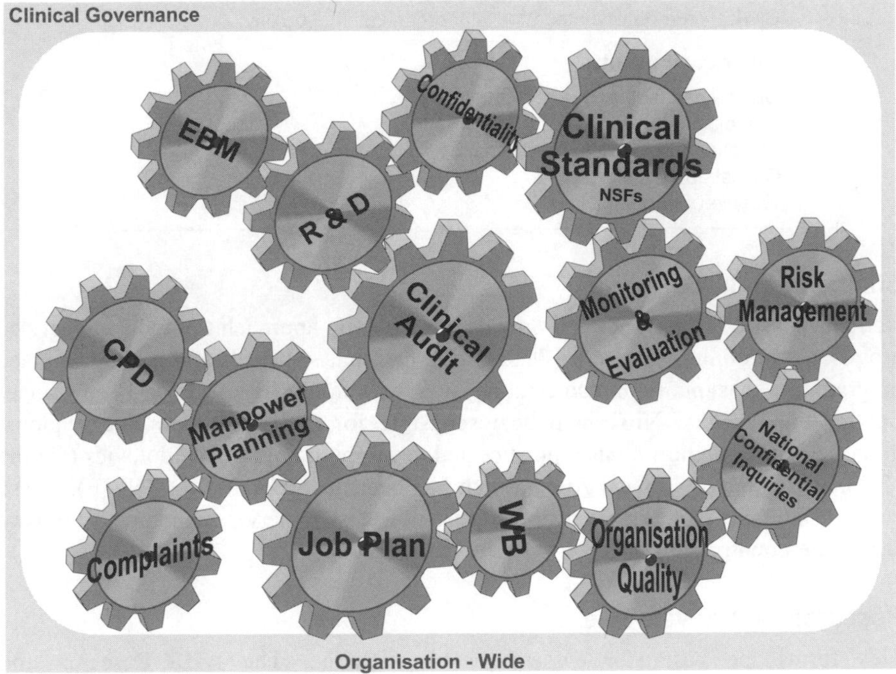

Fig. A1.1 Clinical governance: the system and its components (tools).

improvements where necessary. Many attempts at audit in the past have not gone beyond the setting standards and measuring performance stage. It is imperative that standards and performance are then compared and acted on appropriately. For audit to become user-friendly, trusts and PCGs will need to develop systems to collect high-quality, useful information routinely—a blaming culture must be avoided.

Evidence-based medicine

The white papers make it clear that effective, integrated healthcare must be grounded, where possible, on an evidence base and NICE has been set up to spearhead best practice throughout the NHS. However, much work has already been done by the Cochrane Collaboration, which publishes systematic reviews on healthcare, by the DoH Health Technology Assessment Programme and others.

Table A1.2 Components (tools) of clinical governance

Ten key components:
Clinical audit (individual and service)
National confidential inquiries (eg CEPOD)
Evidence-based medicine (?apply to practice)
Clinical standards (NSFs, NICE, local)
Manpower planning (including retention)
Continuing professional development and lifelong learning
Confidentiality (Caldicott)
Outcome measures (clinical care: individual and service performance)
Research and development (including evaluation of care)
Clinical care quality integrated with organizational quality
Other components:
Clinical risk (self and programme(s))
Complaints
Job plan and individual performance
Critical appraisal
Whistle-blowing

Clinical standards

National service frameworks will provide a systematic approach to models of service provision by defining service models, setting national standards and putting in place programmes to support implementation, and will follow the Calman-Hine Cancer Service Frameworks. NICE will be responsible for appraising new interventions, giving guidance on best clinical practice and developing audit methodologies (via the National Centre for Clinical Audit which has been incorporated into NICE). These clinical standards will help to ensure consistent access to services and quality of care across the country.

Research and development

This forms the basis for evidence-based medicine. The NHS Research and Development Strategy was launched in 1991 to develop a knowledge-based NHS in which decisions (clinical, policy and managerial) would have a sound base. The strategy will continue to have a pivotal role in collecting new evidence, with support from the Horizon Scanning Centre and the National Prescribing Centre in identifying new and existing interventions.

Risk management

Clinical risk reduction programmes and critical incident reporting have been highlighted in the white paper *The New NHS: Modern and Dependable*[(1)] as main components of clinical governance. Clinical risk management aims to achieve four principle objectives:

- proactively to identify areas in which failure might occur and remedy them before failure does occur
- to report incidents when they do occur allowing collection of information for internal investigation and facilitating a speedy settlement if appropriate

- or allowing those involved to learn from their experience
- if all else fails, adequate information will be available for future defence in litigation.

It is important to differentiate between programme risk and individual clinical decision risk assessment.

Monitoring and evaluation

Scrutiny will occur both internally (professional self-regulation, audit) and externally (Commission for Health Improvement, or CHI, the National Survey of Patient and User Experience). The national performance assessment framework has provided the six key areas in which standards should be set and measured:

- health improvement
- fair access
- effectiveness
- efficiency
- patient and carer experiences
- health outcome of NHS care (see Appendix 2).

National confidential inquiries

The four existing national confidential inquiries (into perioperative deaths, stillbirths and deaths in infancy, maternal deaths and suicides) will continue, but will be overseen by NICE.

Job plan and individual performance

This will highlight any areas in the job that are not being met, both presently and as the job develops. Integral to the job plan is continuing professional development.

Continuing professional development (CPD)

This is about developing a culture that encourages lifelong learning (the learning organization) and is an integral part of the job plan. Health organizations should commit, plan and act on 'investment in people' if they are truly interested in delivering quality clinical care.

Complaints

Complaints will be monitored both externally and internally. There will have to be an effective local system in place to deal with complaints. Documentation will be particularly important in order to facilitate external scrutiny.

Manpower planning

This will establish the required staffing levels to achieve acceptable standards of care. However, this is not just about recruiting the appropriate staff, but also about retaining them.

Whistle-blowing

This is to be encouraged. If poorly performing work colleagues are not dealt with/reported, responsibility will be shared. This balance between collective and individual responsibility must be appreciated.

Critical appraisal

Our ability critically to appraise the strength of the evidence available and its application should be part of our routine practice.

Peer-review

Both internal and external peer-review will be an important tool for assessing the effectiveness of the clinical governance culture and in creating a facilitative environment in which excellence can flourish

Figure 1 and the highlight box summarize the key components (tools) of the clinical governance system and the close inter-link between these tools.

Local needs

For clinical governance to be successful, the following must be in place:

- clear lines of responsibility and accountability
- a programme of quality improvement activities
- clear policies aimed at managing risk
- procedures to identify and remedy poor performance.

Statutory requirements

To facilitate the development of clinical governance, the Government has specified the following statutory requirements:

- *health authorities*: to improve the health of their populations
- *trusts*: to improve the quality of services and maintain standards
- *local authorities*: duty of partnership to improve health.

Health authorities in developing a framework for their role in clinical governance have to take into account at least two stands.

- Health authority as a 'health organization'. The easiest way to think about how we all fit into the clinical governance model is to consider duties at each level within the organization, ie the individual, department or directorate, then the organization itself
- Health authority as the 'champion' of the local population. As well as considering clinical governance within its own organization, the health authority needs to fulfil its obligations to the other NHS organizations within its boundaries, namely to facilitate the development of clinical governance within its local trusts and PCGs. To achieve this it must provide support and information and facilitate the exchange of information locally and with other areas. It will also be responsible for monitoring progress by the PCGs.

Table A1.3 Sample terms of reference for a health authority clinical governance committee

Assigning responsibilities for implementation of the committee's recommendations
Providing advice and support to local trusts and PCGs
Monitoring the implementation of clinical governance undertaken by the trusts and PCGs and ensuring they fit in with nationally issued guidance
Ensuring that the problem areas identified have been acted upon appropriately
Implementing and monitoring clinical governance within the health authority
Providing regular reports to the health authority chief executive and to regions
Preparing an annual report for the health authority

To coordinate activities most effectively, a health authority clinical governance committee is proposed. Table A1.3 lists some possible terms of reference for such a committee.

Implementation and costs

While there is a recognition that implementation of clinical governance will require additional resources, it is very difficult to estimate their size and by when they will be needed. Implementation will have to take into account the following principles:

- Good practices that are already in existence and are related to some of the major components (tools) of clinical governance need to be built on
- Quality is not cheap. In some situations there will have to be a balance between quantitative outputs and qualitative clinical outcomes
- Short-term investment in quality improvement leads to long-term gain and may lead to a reduction in unit cost (from a reduction in complications, litigation etc)
- Scrutinizing clinical outcome at the individual level may lead to the practice of defensive medicine by the individual. This can result in excessive numbers of investigations, avoidance of complex or difficult clinical cases, etc. However, clinical risk assessment may help to minimize such defensive practices.

References and further reading

1 Secretary of State for Health. *The new NHS: modern and dependable.* London: The Stationery Office, 1997.
2 Chief Medical Officer. *Clinical governance.* London: DoH, 1999

British Medical Association. *Clinical evidence*, Volume 1. London: BMJ Publishing Group, 1999.
Chalmers I, Altman DG. *Systematic reviews.* London: BMJ Publishing Group, 1995.
Chambers R. *Clinical effectiveness made easy.* Oxford: Radcliffe, 1998.
Department of Health. *A first class service: quality in the new NHS.* London: DoH, 1998.
Gabbey M. *The evidence-based primary care handbook.* London: Royal Society of Medicine Press, 1999.
Gray MJA. *Evidence-based healthcare.* Edinburgh: Churchill Livingstone, 1997.
Harrison S. *Evidence-based medicine: its relevance and application to primary care commissioning.* London: Royal Society of Medicine Press, 1998.
Hopkins A. *Measuring the quality of medical care.* London: The Royal College of Physicians, 1990.
Lugon M, Secker-Walker J. *Clinical governance: making it happen.* London: Royal Society of Medicine Press, 1999.
Scally G, Donaldson LJ. Clinical governance and the drive for quality improvement in the new NHS in England. *Br Med J* 1998; **317**: 61–5.

▸ Appendix 2

National framework for assessing performance in the NHS

Dr Salman Rawaf

Director of Clinical Standards/Senior Lecturer, Merton Sutton and Wandsworth Health Authority, London, UK

Dr Peter Orton

Senior Lecturer, Institute of General Practice, University of Exeter, Exeter, and General Practitioner, Hatfield Heath, UK

The current approach to assessing and managing the performance of the NHS needs to change. A new national framework has been developed to drive improvements in NHS performance and can be used by many different people and organizations. An initial small set of high-level indicators can be used to provide an overview of health authority performance and assess the quality of treatment and care in the new NHS. The plan is to have a robust, broad-based set of indicators covering all areas of the framework. Further development of existing indicators and the development of new indicators will permit a coherent and complementary approach.

The white paper *The New NHS: Modern and Dependable*[(1)] will renew the NHS as a genuinely national service. Patients will get fair access to consistently high quality, prompt and accessible services across the country. The delivery of healthcare against these new national standards will be a matter of local responsibility. Local doctors and nurses will be in the driving seat in shaping services. Stronger links with local authorities will be forged. The needs of the patient will be put at the centre of the care process. Quality will become the driving force for decision-making. This effort should rebuild public confidence in the NHS as a public service.

The new national performance framework will tackle the unacceptable variations that currently exist by comparing performance and sharing best practice, not by financial competition. Benchmarking of performance in different areas and publication of comparative information will allow performance to be compared and best practice shared. The importance of collaborative working across health authorities, local authorities, voluntary organizations and the private sector is recognized.

The new framework sets out for attention the following:

- *health improvement*: to reflect the overarching aim of improving the general health of the population
- *fair access*: to offer fair access to health services in relation to people's needs, irrespective of geography, socioeconomic group, ethnicity, age or sex
- *effective delivery of appropriate healthcare*: to provide care that is effective, appropriate and timely and complies with agreed standards
- *efficiency*: to use NHS resources to achieve value for money

Table A2.1 High-level performance indicators

Areas and categories covered	High-level indicators at health authority level
Health improvement	
Overall health status of populations, reflecting social and environmental factors and individual behavior, as well as care provided by the NHS and other agencies	Deaths from all causes (age 15–64) Deaths from all causes (age 65–74) Cancer registrations
Fair access	
Access to elective surgery	Surgery rates
Access to family services	Conception rates for girls aged 13–15
Access to dentists	Number registered with an NHS dentist
Access to health promotion	Early detection of cancer
Access to community services	District nurse contacts
Effective delivery of appropriate healthcare	
Health promotion/disease prevention	Disease prevention and health promotion Early detection of cancer
Appropriateness of surgery	Inappropriately used surgery Surgery rates
Primary care management	Acute care management Chronic care management Mental health in primary care Cost-effective prescribing
Compliance with standards	Discharge from hospital
Efficiency	
Maximizing use of resources	Day-case rate Length of stay in hospital unit costs Generic prescribing
Patient/carer experience	
Accessibility	Patients who wait >2 hours for emergency admission Patients with operations cancelled for non-medical reasons on the day of or after admission Delayed discharge from hospital for patients aged over 75
Coordination and communication	First outpatient appointments for which patient did not attend
Waiting times	Outpatients seen within 13 weeks of written GP referral Inpatients admitted within 3 months of a decision to admit
Health outcomes of NHS care	
NHS success in reducing level of risk	Conception rate for girls aged 13–15
NHS success in reducing level of impairment and complication of treatment	Decayed, missing and filled teeth in five-year olds Avoidable diseases Adverse events/complications of treatment
NHS success in optimizing function and improving quality of life for patients and carers	Emergency admission to hospital for people aged over 75 Emergency psychiatric readmission
NHS success in reducing premature death	Infant deaths Survival rates for breast and cervical cancer Avoidable deaths Inpatient premature deaths

- *patient/carer experience*: to view the quality of the treatment and care that patients receive and to be sensitive to individual needs
- *health outcomes of NHS care*: to assess the direct contribution of NHS care to improvement in overall health.

A range of different indicator sets will be linked to the framework and available for use by different groups—patients, the public, healthcare professionals, health authorities, primary care groups, NHS trusts and the NHS Executive—both locally and nationally.

To support benchmarking of NHS performance locally and to assess performance across the NHS nationally, a small set of high-level indicators will be developed (Table A2.1). This high-level indicator set aims to give a balanced view of NHS performance at health authority level. Its purpose is to raise questions, highlight areas where further investigation may be required and drive improvements in performance. The indicator set will make use of information already available at health authority level. Some indicators are process measures where measures of outcome, effectiveness and quality are not yet available.

Reference and further reading

1 NHS Executive. *The new NHS: modern and dependable: A national framework for assessing performance.* A consultative document. Leeds: NHSE, 1998.

Department of Health. *A first class service: quality in the new NHS.* London: DoH, 1998.
NHS Executive. *Information for health.* Leeds: NHSE, 1998.

NOTES

NOTES

NOTES